About Island Press

Since 1984, the nonprofit organization Island Press has been stimulating, shaping, and communicating ideas that are essential for solving environmental problems worldwide. With more than 1,000 titles in print and some 30 new releases each year, we are the nation's leading publisher on environmental issues. We identify innovative thinkers and emerging trends in the environmental field. We work with world-renowned experts and authors to develop cross-disciplinary solutions to environmental challenges.

Island Press designs and executes educational campaigns, in conjunction with our authors, to communicate their critical messages in print, in person, and online using the latest technologies, innovative programs, and the media. Our goal is to reach targeted audiences—scientists, policy makers, environmental advocates, urban planners, the media, and concerned citizens—with information that can be used to create the framework for long-term ecological health and human well-being.

Island Press gratefully acknowledges major support from The Bobolink Foundation, Caldera Foundation, The Curtis and Edith Munson Foundation, The Forrest C. and Frances H. Lattner Foundation, The JPB Foundation, The Kresge Foundation, The Summit Charitable Foundation, Inc., and many other generous organizations and individuals.

The opinions expressed in this book are those of the author(s) and do not necessarily reflect the views of our supporters.

Precision Community Health

Berhara

July '22

Precision Community Health

Four Innovations for Well-being

Bechara Choucair

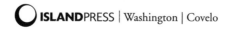

ISLANDPRESS | Washington | Covelo

Library of Congress Control Number: 2019952225

All Island Press books are printed on environmentally responsible materials.

Manufactured in the United States of America
10 9 8 7 6 5 4 3 2 1

Keywords: Affordable Care Act, big data, Centers for Disease Control
(CDC), health disparities, health care, health policy, Healthy Chicago,
housing, Kaiser Permanente, mental health, precision medicine, public
health, teen pregnancy rates, tobacco lobby, vaping

To Mama & Baba: بحبكم *(I love you in Arabic).*
And to three people I love who won't read the book . . . you know who you are!

Contents

Introduction

PUBLIC HEALTH IN THE UNITED STATES IS AT A CROSSROADS. Not simply in terms of the challenges we face to our own well-being, from childhood obesity to lead-tainted water to measles outbreaks, but in the profession itself. Despite a long and storied history, filled with achievements that have fundamentally improved the quality of life of millions of people, the future of public health is far from ensured.

The fact is that the vast majority of people pay no attention to public health issues until a crisis strikes. Tainted water and phony vaccine controversies make headlines, and those headlines flare up into a vigorous but brief debate about how many tax dollars to spend on prevention and treatment. Public health officials such as the head of the Centers for Disease Control and Prevention (CDC) and the surgeon general make the rounds of the talk shows; editorialists editorialize; activists raise the rallying cry. When the crisis passes, as it must, attention moves on. In the meantime, our public health infrastructure, as vital to our national life as our roads and bridges, and in as urgent need of repair, continues to erode.

This is not how things have to be. The future of public health can be bright: it can be a vibrant, innovative field that improves the lives of all who live in this country but especially the overlooked, vulnerable, and disenfranchised—disadvantaged communities; people of color; lesbian, gay, bisexual, and transgender (LGBT) communities; those who are undocumented; and so on. I know because I have seen it happen. That is what this book is about.

Sadly, many public health efforts, while admirably attempting to treat all people equally, have in fact perpetuated a pernicious form of inequality in which the richer you are, the healthier you are. Today, your zip code is as much a determinant of your health as your genetic code. We must become far better at targeting our efforts to those communities that will benefit most from public health innovation.

The goal here is health equity, not equality: we cannot treat all communities in the same way, because their needs are so clearly different. Given the current massive disparities in health across the country, we cannot simply raise all boats on a single tide. To do so would be to continue, perhaps even worsen, the current, and unacceptable, situation.

The time has come for an era of precision community health.

Body, Mind, Community

Health is not just about what happens to us as individuals, to our own bodies, in the physical manifestations of illness. It is also, crucially, about our minds and our communities.

Those physical manifestations have, of course, been the focus of medicine and public health for as long those specialties have existed. Mental health, on the other hand, is quickly rising as a significant concern for physicians and public health officials alike. As the impact and prevalence of depression, anxiety, and other illnesses have become clear, more and more public health agencies have been developing the means to address these issues. But the mind is important to health in more subtle ways. Stress, for example, is a key risk factor in many illnesses, so reducing stress through exercise, access to green spaces in urban areas, and other methods should be part of the public health tool kit.

There is a third piece to the puzzle, in addition to body and mind. That third piece is community. Clearly our health is affected by the physical place and the society in which we live. Do we have access to decent housing? Are our streets safe? Is the air we breathe clean or highly polluted? Can we easily get to a grocery store? These and many other social, environmental, and economic factors play a tangible role in health.

Body, mind, community: that is the framework we can use to help people live the lives they want to live. Once we understand that, we can begin to use all the tools of modern technology to get there. Medical science is getting more precise every day. *Precision medicine*, the phrase itself, was coined by Western Australia's Office of Population Health Genomics and refers to targeting treatments to individuals on the basis of genetic differences. Precision medicine offers the prospect of customized, effective treatment for a wide variety of ailments. It garnered wide attention in the United States in 2015, when President Barack Obama unveiled his $215 million Precision Medicine Initiative. President Obama called precision medicine "one of the greatest opportunities for new medical breakthroughs that we have ever seen," saying that it promised to deliver "the right treatments at the right time, every time, to the right person."

Precision public health is the idea of applying those techniques across populations, offering new insights into who is at risk of which illnesses and what can be done to prevent them.[1] Muin J. Khoury, head of the CDC's Office of Genomics and Precision Public Health, has described this term in academic papers and blogs.

That is a powerful idea. It is also a limited one. Applying a medical model to public health may indeed lead to improvements, but it may also miss the key insights of the body, mind, community framework. This is where precision community health comes in. *Precision community health* involves taking advantage of new tools, including cutting-edge data and communication technologies, and using traditional methods, such as coalition building, in new ways to target public health interventions in the most effective way possible. Doing so will help people access healthy meals, affordable homes, safe playgrounds, and supportive schools. That is what I mean by precision community health.

This is fundamentally an optimistic story. It is about improving public health for the people who need it most, in the most challenging circumstances. There is compelling evidence that this new approach can produce dramatic results. I saw them in Chicago, where I served as commissioner of public health from 2009 to 2014, and I see them now on a broader scale in my position as chief community health officer at Kaiser Permanente. In Chicago, reductions in smoking rates, teen births, and breast cancer mortality happened as a result of the hard work of so many people in our communities working together tirelessly in the spirit of precision community health.

If we want to see those results replicated, public health practitioners and policy makers must choose to take the field in a new direction. Otherwise it will wither into irrelevance, with public responsibilities devolved to private institutions that might not be suited to meeting the needs of diverse and growing urban populations. And those needs are critical. In too many communities, poor health has become the norm.

I grew up in an extreme example of poor community health: Lebanon in the midst of a civil war. I saw how violence hurt individuals, neighborhoods, and the whole country. I suffered from violence myself. I saw how it changed my own family.

In medical school at the American University of Beirut, I spent time seeing patients in Palestinian refugee camps. I talked to so many people who lived their whole lives in an environment where I would never want to live. I saw the devastation caused by forced migration.

During my training in family medicine at Baylor College of Medicine in Houston, Texas, and then as medical director of Crusader Community Health, a community health center network in Rockford, Illinois, I met migrant families, people in need of public housing, and those living with HIV/AIDS. Working in these places taught me how poverty shapes both communities and individuals.

What I learned from all these experiences is simple: health is about far more than health care alone. We also have to think about housing. We have to think about economic security. We have to think about legal protections. This is what precision community health is all about.

Health equity boils down to this: Are we creating an environment where vulnerable people can have the best chance for healthy lives? Getting to that point will mean changing the built environment, the policies, and the public health strategies that either are standing in the way of health equity or are insufficient to the task at hand.

The key will be found in applying twenty-first-century technology, along with sound policies and savvy understanding of the modern media landscape, to solving the problems that have long challenged public health officials. It will also mean deeply listening to communities that have until now been neglected and working with people in those communities to design solutions. Both municipal and state governments need to embrace new methods. If they don't, the profession of public health as we know it will become obsolete.

Far from something to be taken up after we have reduced the deficit or changed the tax structure, this new approach to health provides a sound foundation for everything else. The payoff for the investment in precision community health that we make now will be nothing less than thriving cities and communities for generations to come.

Where We've Been and Where We Are Going

During my time in Chicago I saw public health move from the shadows at the end of Mayor Richard Daley's long tenure to the forefront of Mayor Rahm Emanuel's agenda for the city. And I saw the combination of twenty-first-century technology with good, old-fashioned community building.

This blending of the old and the new has brought us to the edge of an exciting era. What we will see over the next five to ten years, I believe, will be the era of precision community health: crafting solutions to health challenges that are tailored to the needs of specific communities through the innovative use of technology, public policy, media, and deep community engagement. These innovations could not come at a more fitting moment.

Congress periodically becomes embroiled in fierce debates over how much money to spend on combating whatever crisis is currently in the headlines. Lost in the blur of numbers are three more pressing questions. First, can we predict where the next outbreak, the next crisis, will be? Anticipating, rather than simply responding to, crises is the next leap for improving public health in the United States and around the world. Second, once we have anticipated a crisis, can we act effectively to combat it? Third, and most important, what can we do to prevent a crisis from happening in the first place? Those are the questions that precision community health must solve.

The long history of public health in Chicago shows how far we have come and how far we still have to go. Just as it does today, in 1832 a sense of crisis drove the city to act. Troops on their way to the Black Hawk War brought cholera to Chicago, helping to spread what was already a worldwide pandemic. Five years later, Chicago's charter created the Board of Health and the position of health officer. Over the next century, the city took on such challenges as diphtheria, scarlet and typhoid fevers, measles, and whooping cough, as well as the health problems caused by the meatpacking industry and other industries. Chicago cleaned its water supply and began efforts to address the needs of the working poor.

Only government could have achieved results at that scale. Indeed, the history of public health in Chicago and in other US cities is a testament to the irreplaceable role that government at all levels must play in improving health. But that history, as well as current experience, points out the limitations of what government can accomplish on its own.

We are now on the verge of what Lester Breslow, one of the true giants of public health, called the third revolution. Chicago's history provides clear examples of the first revolution, addressing communicable disease, and the second, making progress in treating chronic disease. The third revolution, in which the goal is health and health equity rather than just disease prevention, may be the most challenging yet the most rewarding of them all.

The third revolution will require a social movement, a shift in public attitudes about what constitutes public health. To promote health, we need to think beyond clinical medicine. We have to be involved in social policy, fiscal policy, education, and housing. All of these bear, directly and indirectly, on health.

The third revolution also requires an understanding of what the private sector can and cannot do. There is a trend, spurred in part by the success of the Affordable Care Act, to shift public health responsibilities to the private sector. More and more expertise is moving from government agencies to corporate enterprises. Some might even think that the private sector can take on that role on its own. What is needed is not a wholesale shift of public to private but a far deeper collaboration between health care and public health. Indeed, Tom Frieden, who was director of the CDC and hence the nation's top public health officer under President Obama, said that strengthening that collaboration will be the top challenge for public health over the next decade.

Public health needs to step up and reclaim its rightful place, not just as the last line of defense against the next crisis but as the profession best suited to ensuring healthy communities far into the future. The window of opportunity for public health practitioners and policy makers to demonstrate their continued relevance is narrow, but it remains open.

If public health is to take advantage of that opportunity, it will need to evolve, and quickly. The history of public health has been of gradual change over the course of decades as new challenges emerged and new approaches emerged to combat them. That pattern cannot continue. Public health needs a jump start, something that both solves pressing problems and reestablishes the field as something worthy of our best minds and increased public funding and support.

The Four Pillars of Precision Community Health

During my tenure as Chicago's commissioner of public health I saw firsthand how public health is changing. The lessons I learned during that time are broadly applicable to other cities and are relevant to anyone interested in new ways to meet the persistent and, indeed, growing challenges of our complex metropolises.

The stakes are high. Traditional efforts have fallen short because dismaying trajectories have not changed—poor communities continue to suffer disproportionately from scourges such as childhood obesity, diabetes, smoking, and HIV/AIDS. But we have at our fingertips the data and technologies we need, as well as a better understanding of the connections between social justice, economic prosperity, and health.

Big cities will continue to be centers of innovation, and now is the time to invest in their efforts. Governments are starting to adopt strategies to use big data and analytics to improve public health. The jurisdictions implementing these practices give an enticing glimpse of the technology's potential and a sense of the challenges that stand in the way. This is a rapidly evolving environment, and cities can work with partners such as civic tech communities, health-care systems, and emerging markets to introduce new methods for solving old problems.

Precision community health rests on four pillars: big data, policy, media, and coalition building. Some are familiar, some innovative, but all need to be employed in a new way if they are to become the foundation of a better approach to public health challenges. The advent of radically improved computing and communication technologies and new ways of serving long-neglected communities offers dramatic possibilities.

Big Data

Precision community health is just the jump start we need. Translating data into actionable knowledge is the challenge for a new generation of civic-minded public health and community leaders if we are serious about improving people's lives. It is a way to reinvigorate the profession and to take advantage of the enormous opportunity to prevent, rather than simply respond to, public health crises. The fact is that public health has for too long been seen as a stodgy backwater. Designing apps that make it easy for people to find birth control, report a public health problem, and interact with local health offices is one way to demonstrate that public health has entered the twenty-first century.

The need for new approaches is clear in one of the most traditional and visible public health functions: restaurant inspections. To keep Chicago's fifteen thousand food establishments safe, in the early part of the twentieth century the city was divided into districts, each headed by a supervising sanitarian, with a team of food sanitarians who rotated across the districts and inspected every restaurant once per year or responded to reports of problems. Even the title *sanitarian* reflects the roots of urban health initiatives in nineteenth-century ideas of public hygiene. We can do better.

So, in 2013, we added a new approach. We identified various data related to food establishments and their locations—building code violations, sourcing of food, registered complaints, lighting in alleys behind food establishments, nearby construction, social media reports, sanitation code violations, neighborhood population density, complaint histories of other establishments with the same owner, and more. Those data led to an algorithm that produced a risk score for every food establishment, with higher risk scores associated with a greater likelihood of identifying critical violations.

Then we did the same thing with lead toxicity and built a predictive model using two decades of blood lead level tests, home lead inspections, property value assessments, and census data. We identified units where the risk was highest in order to prevent lead exposure before it happens. From ensuring clean water supplies to delivering polio vaccines, the most effective public health interventions help avert crises before they start. However, predicting the next crisis has always proven a challenge for the profession. Predictive analytics enables public health officials to concentrate their efforts, leading to better outcomes and lower costs.

That promise can also be seen at Kaiser Permanente, which has been collecting data for decades and has been a data-driven organization since its founding. In 2016, Kaiser Permanente launched a five-year, $13 million study to revisit data collected in the early years of the organization to evaluate how risk factors in early life and midlife have affected brain health and dementia risk among a large, ethnically diverse cohort of seniors. In particular, researchers aim to explore how early-life conditions may play a role in racial and ethnic differences in dementia rates and risk factors for cognitive decline, an area that has not been well studied.

Kaiser Permanente has a long track record of applying data in clinical settings, and the systems have evolved to the point at which physicians know which hospitalized patients are at risk of ending up in the intensive care unit and which members are likely to need the most health services down the line. We are also exploring how the same approach translates to improving community health. The potential impact is evident. For example, the wealth of clinical data we have about our patients, coupled with publicly available data, may help us develop strategies to prevent people from becoming homeless or to address food insecurity for pregnant women.

Policy

Precision community health is not just about data and technology. We can also be far more precise in the policies we create.

Big Tobacco learned the value of precision long ago, to the detriment of public health. Tobacco companies have become immensely skilled at getting their deadly products into just the right hands at just the right age. That usually means targeting disadvantaged communities and getting people hooked as young as possible. We need to learn those lessons too if we are to level the playing field in the public interest.

In Chicago we took a targeted approach to the tobacco problem. The first step was to raise the price of cigarettes through taxes. We had a simple rule: you can never raise cigarette taxes enough. I am proud to say that today Chicago has the highest cigarette tax anywhere. A pack of cigarettes in Chicago costs twelve dollars, more than seven dollars of which goes back to the city and the state in the form of taxes.

This is not simply a matter of raising taxes for the sake of raising taxes. Raising the price of cigarettes impacts those who are the most price-sensitive consumers: children and adolescents, the groups that need the most support in ensuring that they don't pick up that first cigarette.

The second step was to regulate the sale of tobacco and tobacco products near schools. The city banned the sale of flavored tobacco, including menthol-flavored tobacco, within 500 feet of schools. Finally, and way before e-cigarettes became so popular, we knew we had to address the new set of problems that they would bring to our communities. If it is not okay for a twelve-year-old to purchase cigarettes, the same should be true for e-cigarettes, which are just another way to get kids hooked on nicotine at an early age. So we raised the minimum age, first to eighteen and then to twenty-one. We also required vendors to have a license to sell e-cigarettes and required them to keep e-cigarettes behind the counter.

We must think and act systemically if we want to create real change. That is as true for local issues as it is for far broader challenges. At Kaiser

Permanente, for example, we believe that mitigating climate change is a key component of our community health agenda in order to prevent illness and safeguard the health of people everywhere. Shifting from fossil fuels to renewable power creates immediate public health benefits because it reduces air pollution, and that lowers the risk for asthma and other respiratory diseases. Walking, cycling, and taking public transit instead of driving reduces chronic diseases and air pollution. As the nation's largest nonprofit integrated health-care system, Kaiser Permanente has a responsibility to support health at every opportunity, including efforts to reduce and eliminate the environmental causes of illness.

When its environmental stewardship work began twenty years ago, Kaiser Permanente focused on getting mercury and other hazardous materials out of medical supplies, such as intravenous equipment, and building materials. More recently, we called on suppliers to eliminate toxic flame retardants and introduced safer cleaning systems to protect patients and workers. Today, we look across our entire organization and ask how we can improve community health and reduce the considerable environmental footprint of the health-care sector and its supply chains. That kind of systemic thinking has created an extremely powerful vision for Kaiser Permanente as an organization.

Media

Another key element of Chicago's approach to tobacco illustrates how precision community health can play out. Just as Big Tobacco used the media to create its toxic brands, we needed to learn how to use the media to reveal the far more troubling side of those slick images.

First, we realized that with so many ways to get information, we would need something dramatic to cut through the media clutter. We would need to push the envelope as hard as we could.

We developed an ad campaign that targeted African American lesbians in Chicago, a community with one of the highest smoking rates in the city. One of the ads featured an image of two women kissing, a first for a public service ad in Chicago, and it raised some eyebrows when we placed it on the sides of city buses. We also posted those ads in gay bars around the city. And they got people talking. In one set of ads to raise awareness about teenage pregnancy, we had images of "pregnant" teen boys. We wanted the ads to be provocative. We wanted those images to spark conversation, and that's exactly what happened. The ads generated international news coverage and a flurry of social media attention.

The lessons we learned from that targeted approach are now being applied elsewhere. A campaign called Action Minded developed by Kaiser Permanente and the Public Good Projects (PGP), a nonprofit organization focused on using modern communication technology to change behavior. The idea behind this campaign is to reduce the stigma associated with mental illness and to increase awareness about mental health.

Several weeks after launching this campaign we saw a great response, with more than twenty thousand followers, nineteen million impressions, and four hundred thousand engagements. The campaign is on track to becoming the largest mental health anti-stigma campaign ever, one that is taking precision community health to the next level.

The PGP harnesses data from across mainstream and social media to develop historical, real-time, and predictive analytics regarding mental health stigma in the United States. For example, in a first for any public health behavior change campaign, the individuals highlighted in one component of the campaign are identified exclusively from this media monitoring. This is precision marketing in action and in service to the public welfare.

Coalition Building
Precision community health can also help shape the way we think about how to build coalitions and to what end. The effort I helped develop

with Mayor Emanuel, called Healthy Chicago, was anchored in a deep commitment to community engagement.

In Healthy Chicago, we focused our efforts on those who are most disenfranchised and supported them in lifting themselves up. It was not about lifting everyone, at least not at first. We took a social justice approach, and that's why we targeted menthol in cigarettes, teen pregnancy among blacks and Latinos, and so on. With so many challenges, we felt compelled to target the neediest communities first. That may seem obvious, but it is not the way public health has always worked.

For one thing, local governments typically focus on three fundamental responsibilities: safety, education, and jobs. If time and money are left over for other things, fine, but those three rank far above everything else. Mayor Emanuel was different: when he took office, he was determined to raise the profile of public health. So my challenge was to find ways to make that happen in the most effective ways possible.

Mayor Emanuel had a checklist of the things he wanted to get done in his first one hundred days in office. We both agreed that developing a public health agenda for the city needed to be on that list. On the ninety-seventh day of the administration, at a meeting with community partners, we launched Healthy Chicago.

To get there, we needed to deeply engage the community. Fortunately, during my brief tenure under Mayor Daley, I had begun to learn the nitty-gritty of Chicago politics and how nothing can replace face-to-face communication. Chicago is full of legends about ward heelers and aldermen, but they were on to something vital: getting anything done in Chicago means getting out into the streets and learning what people really want from their government.

Early on in my tenure as commissioner, I set a simple rule: no community meeting was too small, too late in the day, or too far away for me to attend. My team would ask me why I was going, for example, to a meeting of a small group of mothers on the South Side. The simple answer was "Because they asked." I was building relationships as well as accumulating social capital that I suspected I would have to spend one day, when tough decisions would have to be made. It turned out that I was right about that. The advent of precision community health does not relieve officials of the responsibility to make those decisions, but it can clarify the decisions. Part of what this book is about is exploring when we can turn to new technologies for insight and when we must rely on our own judgment and insight and the wisdom of the communities we serve.

Building coalitions does not necessarily generate headlines. Generally, politicians don't get to cut red ribbons at the opening of a gleaming new partnership. Coalition building requires the day-in, day-out work of countless public health professionals across the country, and it can be slow, frustrating, and exhausting. But it is also essential. Together with the community, we were able to codesign and launch innovative efforts in Chicago. Some of them generated nationwide coverage and, occasionally, some controversy. But none would have been possible had we not laid the foundation first.

We are seeing the same thing at Kaiser Permanente. The Healthy Eating Active Living (HEAL) Cities Campaign is a nationwide collaboration launched by Kaiser Permanente and involving dozens of local governments and organizations. The campaign works to advance health equity by passing policy resolutions for general plans, land use, healthy food access, and work-site wellness. Over the past seven years, the campaign has worked with 305 cities with more than 19 million residents. The effort has helped craft more than one thousand policies that have been adopted and collaborated with more than 2,300 elected officials.

These four pillars—big data, policy, media, and coalition building—support a new way of approaching the health challenges of our communities. Building on them will demand changes in how public health officials and organizations think, are trained, and interact with the public at large. Such change is never easy, but it is both welcome and essential. To understand why, we need first to look back at where public health began, as its roots offer insight into both the aspects of the field that should change and those that should not.

CHAPTER 1

Public Health in Chicago and Beyond

In the United States, we tend to believe that our health is largely a result of our genes and our personal choices. But research shows that health is also influenced by our environment. That's what led me to a career in public health: if we can improve the health of a neighborhood, we can improve the health of its residents.

Soon after I immigrated to the United States in 1997, I started training to become a family physician in a program focused on caring for people living in poverty and facing homelessness, many of whom were also immigrants. In the beginning I was optimistic, full of hope that my medical training would provide all that my patients needed to optimize their health.

After I completed my residency and was working in Rockford, Illinois, I met Judy. She was charming and engaging and always had a story to tell. She was in her mid-thirties.

On the surface, her ailments were straightforward: aches and pains, minor infections, and some obvious symptoms of her years of substance abuse. But as we talked more, it became clear that her challenges ran deeper. Her mental health issues got in the way of her holding down a job, and her chronic unemployment made it impossible for her to get the right health care. The care I could provide wasn't ever going to break this vicious cycle. The help she needed wasn't going to come from within the walls of a clinic.

I felt powerless. These weren't symptoms they covered in medical school. So what happens when "Do no harm" doesn't feel like enough because what you really want is to "do the most good"?

One afternoon in the clinic with Judy gave me the answer. As usual, we discussed her health issues: anxiety, depression, and addiction. Then she told me what she was really worried about: finding a place to sleep on those frigid winter nights in Illinois and whether or not she'd freeze to death.

In our clinics, we worked closely with social service agencies to try to connect folks like Judy with resources, but it never felt like enough. Each time Judy left, we both knew there was a chance she wouldn't come back. One day, I got word that someone had died from hypothermia in a park near the clinic. When I learned it was Judy, it broke my heart. Her death had been preventable, but prevention was out of my reach. I felt I had failed her. Our systems had failed her. Our community had failed her.

I couldn't write a prescription to treat homelessness. Helping the Judys of the world would require broadening my practice from individuals to communities. We have to support entire populations, the systems that impact them, and the places in which they live. I shifted my focus from patients to policies, from office hours to organizational impact. And I began looking for partners in my new "practice," recognizing that no doctor could do it alone.

A community-level focus means seeing populations as a whole, which is where sophisticated technology comes in, helping to collect and analyze data more efficiently. We are already seeing the possibilities in action. In October 2018, the US Census Bureau, in collaboration with researchers at Harvard and Brown Universities, published nation-wide data that for the first time will make it possible to pinpoint where children of all backgrounds have the best shot at success.[1] And *pinpoint* is precisely what I mean: according to the research, children are most affected by what happens within about one-half mile of their homes. For years we knew about neighborhood disparities—in a city such as Chicago it is painfully apparent—but the fine details were missing because we did not have the capacity to sift through all the data. Now we can, and this makes real the promise of big data, as it offers the opportunity to get to the root of neighborhood disadvantage.

This is the kind of advance that makes precision community health possible. But it is more than a question of computing power and sophisticated algorithms. Before we could even consider the technical details, we needed a fundamental shift in perspective. For years we thought that health was only what happened in our bodies. It is no surprise, then, that the field of public health has traditionally been focused on medicine. As a physician myself, I am reminded daily of the invaluable insights that medicine offers to public health.

Yet there is obviously more to treating illness than understanding particular bodily systems. Over the past decade or so, more and more professionals have begun to recognize not only the second piece of the puzzle, mental health, but also the third: community.

Rahm Emanuel understood the power of the body, mind, community approach to public health. When he was elected mayor of Chicago in 2011, he directed the Chicago Department of Public Health (CDPH) to create a comprehensive agenda for the entire city. We called it Healthy Chicago.[2] Our vision was quite simple: identify specific areas of health that need improvement and tackle these issues in an effective and accountable way. As a result, we identified twelve priorities to address through policy, programs, and public education, all of which can be monitored and measured.

The choice of the title was no accident. We wanted to focus not on healthy Chicagoans but on healthy Chicago. That is where we believed health starts, happens, and evolves. In fact, most of what affects health has nothing to do with our behavior—it is related to social factors such as our education, employment, and family situation, as well as environmental factors such as housing and air quality, along with access to quality medical care.[3] How can you think about being healthy if you don't know where you're going to sleep or get a meal or how you will get paid? How can students think about homework—since education is key to getting and staying out of poverty—if they're hungry? What you actually do, such as exercise, refrain from smoking, eat a healthy diet, and so on, is absolutely relevant but is not the main driver of health.

In retrospect, our plan seems like plain common sense. But it was quite a departure from the way public health has traditionally been approached. The history of public health in the United States, and in Chicago in particular, shows that while we have indeed made great strides, we still have a long way to go. In fact, we see history repeating itself in many current controversies over environmental justice, regulation of businesses, and the routine vaccination of children. All these issues have telling historical parallels and are playing out now in ways that are eerily similar to what happened a century or two ago.

The fundamental goal of the public health field has not changed since its earliest days in the American colonies: to protect individuals and communities from disease and other threats to their welfare. In the nineteenth century, containing the spread of infectious diseases such as smallpox and yellow fever was central to that mission. Those two scourges could sweep across communities with devastating speed and force, which made them the focus of early public health efforts. Other diseases, such as tuberculosis, malaria, and dysentery, actually caused far more deaths, but they were slow-moving and familiar, common burdens to be borne or punishments from God that demanded prayer and fasting, not community action. The unfamiliar, however, especially if it seemed to come from outside the community, dominated the public imagination.

The same is still true today. Outbreaks of rare diseases generate global headlines. The ravages of Ebola, dengue fever, or even the occasional case of bubonic plague are indeed frightening, but they cause relatively few deaths compared with, say, smoking, or heart disease that stems from poor diet and lack of exercise. Addressing those deep-seated problems means taking on questions of lifestyle, behavior, and poverty, issues that were not considered part of public health until the late nineteenth and early twentieth centuries, when the scope of the field quickly began to widen. Disease is not simply a biophysical process, a question of infectious agents, vectors, and hosts, but also a social one. Nearly everything people do within a community—how and where they live, where they work, how they interact with their neighbors—has a bearing, either direct or indirect, on their likelihood of becoming ill or staying healthy. That understanding has emerged gradually but now is key to the idea of precision community health.

Crisis, Response, Complacency

Precision community health also uses new tools to break an entrenched cycle in public health practice: a health crisis emerges; physicians, communities, businesses, and governments respond; the crisis fades from memory. Lather, rinse, repeat. A good part of this is human nature: we are often motivated to dramatic action only in the face of imminent danger. Maintaining that level of effort over the long term is expensive, exhausting, and sometimes counterproductive. But the pattern also has social and cultural roots that reach back to the early European settlers in North America.

For colonial cities such as Boston, Philadelphia, and Charleston, the first priority was to keep potential sources of infection off their shores. By the turn of the eighteenth century, both Boston and Charleston required ships arriving from infected ports or with sick passengers aboard to submit to inspection and transfer the sick to "pesthouses" located offshore.[4]

As trade expanded, so did the use of quarantine laws across the colonies. But as the fears of a particular disease outbreak faded, so did the vigilance in enforcing the laws. Then a new outbreak would emerge, and the public outcry would lead to new, tougher laws. That dynamic remains a challenge for improving public health, as any far-reaching efforts require persistent attention from communities and elected officials alike, and that attention always seems fleeting. One of the strengths of a precision approach to public health is that it targets specific issues within specific communities, where maintaining attention may be more feasible than across large and diverse cities or states.

That approach also has the potential to address two other public health challenges with deep historical roots: dirty and dangerous industries are often concentrated in poor communities, and enforcing public health laws is seen as an affront to unfettered capitalism and personal liberty. Both issues are at the forefront of public health debates today, just as they were in the eighteenth and nineteenth centuries.

In 1793, the first in a series of devastating yellow fever epidemics swept from Boston to New Orleans and everywhere in between. More epidemics came in the years that followed. According to historian John Duffy, the years between 1793 and 1806 deserve to be called the yellow fever era.[5] The disease hit Philadelphia first, then Baltimore, New Haven, and New York. Both Philadelphia and New York used groups of citizen volunteers to organize a response to the crisis. Eventually New York created a formal Health Committee and gave it broad, if temporary, powers.

Among the issues the Health Committee took on was the overall cleanliness of the city. The concern was based on the prevailing theory at the time, which attributed disease to a gaseous substance called miasma, thought to emanate from stagnant water and putrefying matter. The miasmatic theory would of course eventually be shown to be completely false, but it spurred widespread efforts to keep cities clean. Following a 1798 yellow fever outbreak in New York, the city commissioned a report that linked the disease to nearly every sanitation issue of the day, from damp cellars to smelly pickled fish to narrow lanes.[6]

Concerns over sanitation would shape public health efforts for decades. Previously, cleanliness had been largely a question of aesthetics for colonial towns and cities. Keeping garbage and sewage from fouling the streets made daily life far more pleasant, but no one made the connection to actual physical well-being. As cities grew, the stench caused by so-called nuisance industries—slaughterhouses, tanneries, bone-boiling and fat-rendering establishments—forced town officials to relocate them, though with reluctance because it was usually the poor who were forced to live nearby. That pattern, too, would be repeated time and again, and it continues to pose a significant challenge to public health efforts and the lives of impoverished communities in many parts of the world.

There were, and continue to be, major obstacles to sanitation. The first is entrenched economic interests, as well as powerful American ideals of liberty and free enterprise. It is far cheaper for an industry to dump waste into the nearest stream or vacant lot in the poorest quarter of town than to design and implement methods to dispose of it properly. Businesses do not want to be told to move or how to maintain their property, or have their goods stuck on a ship that cannot be unloaded because of quarantine. The roots of today's opposition to government regulation of business run deep indeed.

But it is not just businesses that resist any limits on their freedom to do as they choose, when they choose. City residents also have a stubborn resistance to being told what to do with their trash, despite endless and creative efforts to convince them not to toss it in the street. One need only walk around any major city to know that cleanliness does not come naturally to groups of people living together, and it probably never has.

Yellow fever forced people to take dramatic steps, such as forming health boards that cared for the sick and the poor while improving living conditions for all. But then the epidemic passed, and so did the energy required to bring lasting change. Between the 1790s and 1830, with the single exception of Boston's, every health board created to respond to public health crises was temporary.[7] While the idea that government action was required to protect public health may have been born during the yellow fever era, it would not be a permanent part of American life for some time to come.

A Role for Government

People only slowly recognized that when it came to something as fundamental as protecting communities from deadly disease epidemics, there were some steps that no volunteer effort, no matter how organized and effective, could take. In truth, the quarantines and cleanup efforts spurred by yellow fever outbreaks did little to control the spread of the disease, since it is spread by mosquitoes, which respond only indirectly to improvements in hygiene, unlike, say, salmonella. While this may have had some side benefits, real progress against disease would require a combination of better science and effective government. The opportunity for both soon presented itself in the form of a transformational medical advance that has saved countless lives and should not be the least bit controversial, yet somehow today has become a flash point for the ugliest and most destructive of debates: vaccination.

Smallpox was by far the most feared disease in colonial America, and for good reason. It was a horrific malady. A seemingly healthy person would suddenly develop a high fever, headache, and backache. She or he would start to vomit and become delirious. By the third or fourth day of such suffering, things would get even worse as red spots would appear on the face and around the eyes, and these would soon turn to pus-filled blisters. Smallpox killed 20 to 40 percent of its victims. Even if the patient survived, the blisters would leave permanent, disfiguring scars and even blindness. In the seventeenth and eighteenth centuries, one-third of the population of London bore smallpox scars.[8]

Smallpox had plagued humanity for millennia, and for just as long, healers had searched for cures. Arab and Chinese physicians knew by at least the eighteenth century and probably far earlier that people who survived the disease became immune to further infection, at least for a time, and so they came up with the idea of provoking a mild case of smallpox by making small incisions in a healthy person's arm and rubbing material gleaned from a smallpox blister into them. The subject in most cases developed a mild case of smallpox and became immune to the disease.[9]

The procedure was called inoculation or sometimes variolation, from the Latin word for smallpox, *variola*. It was effective but far from perfect: more than 10 percent of those inoculated died. While lower than the mortality from the disease itself, such a high rate of complications meant that widespread acceptance of the procedure was slow in coming, despite the enthusiastic endorsement of many physicians. Nevertheless, inoculation brought at least a measure of control over smallpox in the United States by the turn of the nineteenth century.

By that time a better alternative was already available. An English physician named Edward Jenner had heard stories that milkmaids who caught cowpox—a harmless disease that affected the udders and teats of cows—on their hands never developed smallpox. In 1796, Jenner made two small incisions on the arm of an eight-year-old boy named James Phipps, son of a homeless laborer. He dipped his lancet first into the cowpox lesions on the hands of a local girl and then into the incisions. After eight days, James developed pustules similar to those of cowpox and a slight fever, but both soon faded. A month after the initial procedure, Jenner variolated Phipps, which should have produced a mild case of smallpox. Yet no such symptoms appeared. Jenner had for the first time demonstrated that giving a healthy person a mild disease could protect them from a far more devastating one, and the vaccine was born.[10]

Some American physicians clung to the older method of inoculation, requiring new laws in some cases to prohibit vaccination. Then, in 1809, the town of Milton, Massachusetts, embarked on a campaign to vaccinate all of its residents against smallpox. It was so successful that it led the state to vaccinate all residents, at public expense. Compliance was voluntary and therefore the law had relatively little practical effect, but it was a watershed moment. Four years later, at the urging of Thomas Jefferson, Congress passed the first federal law to encourage vaccination. The principle that government should be involved in public health issues, and that it should take particular interest in the health of the poor, was ever more firmly established in the public mind.[11]

The flip side of that principle was, however, just as firmly entrenched: government should be involved in public health issues only in times of crisis. That idea led to the repeal of the federal vaccine law about a decade after it was passed. And the pattern of crisis, response, complacency too often remains the defining feature of public health efforts in the United States.

There are echoes of the early debates about vaccination in the current controversy. As is the case today, while the vast majority of physicians quickly saw the importance of Jenner's discovery, a minority never came around and clung to the old ways, and a portion of the general public agreed. And as also is the case today, governments were forced to embark on public education campaigns to convince skeptics that vaccines were both safe and effective.

There is another, more troubling parallel as well. Most of the early health boards in cities such as Boston, New York, and Philadelphia consisted entirely of laypeople. No physicians were appointed because there was a general distrust of the medical profession. The raging debates among doctors about the cause of disease convinced many people that in a crisis the doctors would be so divided they would be unable to take action.[12] Today, that distrust—particularly of pharmaceutical manufacturers but of physicians as well—still echoes across social media–driven conspiracy theories about vaccines.

The distrust of doctors faded but never disappeared entirely, even though for many decades the status of doctors in society was nearly unassailable. Vaccination became almost universally accepted and led to extinction of the smallpox virus—save for a few samples held in high-security research facilities—and the near-total control of once widespread diseases such as polio and measles. The trajectory of progress seemed fixed, but the advent of mass communication technology, and with it the ability to spread misinformation and outright falsehoods, changed that. The fact that there is today a small but vocal group of opponents to vaccination, falling vaccination rates in some communities, and a concomitant rise in entirely preventable diseases, particularly measles, marks a dramatic step back toward the nineteenth century. Public health professionals have been slow to adopt modern communication tools. We have to change that.

Sanitarians and the Roots of Precision

The Industrial Revolution brought with it a host of opportunities and challenges to American cities. Working conditions, especially among the poor, were horrific. In Europe, that led to calls for broad reform and the eventual creation of national boards of health. But reform was slow to come in the United States. One reason, argues historian John Duffy, was that the urgency of the abolition movement understandably absorbed all the energy of reformers. Faced with such a momentous fight, they had little attention left for issues of public health.

Efforts to improve public health in the United States were local and sporadic, with no organized national effort and little even at state levels.

Some cities, such as Boston, took progressive steps. Others did little or nothing until catastrophe was upon them. Individual cities were driven to respond to epidemics but were nearly paralyzed by the inability of medical science at the time either to explain the causes of those epidemics or to treat the victims effectively. With the miasmatic theory still firmly in place, the focus remained on urging residents to remove the carcasses of their dead animals from the streets and to refrain from building new privies in city centers.

It was largely a losing battle. Streets filled with rubbish, blood from slaughterhouses ran in the gutters, and almost any ditch or stream became an open sewer. City governments struggled to gain a foothold as the populations boomed. With little capacity or willingness to regulate who lived where, and in what conditions, cities ended up overcrowded, with new arrivals relegated to ramshackle dwellings, often in low-lying, poorly drained areas. The urban slum, among the most persistent and refractory problems in public health, has been a fixture of the American landscape for nearly two centuries.

Access to clean water was a particular concern. Cities such as Philadelphia and Baltimore began installing lead pipes to carry water to their residents by the 1820s, but the idea of filtering or treating water was years away. As cities grew, their water sources became polluted and water quality deteriorated steadily.[13] Even in the best of circumstances, only the wealthiest had water in their homes; everyone else waited in line by public wells or bought river water from water carriers. For the poor, living in crowded conditions with little or no sanitation, the situation was far direr, but without the drama of the yellow fever epidemics to spur public action, little was done.

Two developments began to change that dynamic. One was subtle; the other was anything but. The subtle change came from a deepening appreciation of the kinds of insights that could come from applying statistics to questions of public health. Up until the early nineteenth century, governments collected statistics only for the purpose of assessing the size of the population or measuring economic activity, particularly trade. The word *statistics* itself, introduced in English only in 1787, referred to the collection of information of interest to the state. Since health conditions were of only fleeting interest to the state—when yellow fever or smallpox epidemics were nigh, for example—few people saw the need to collect different kinds of information, and fewer still would have known what to do with the information once they had it.

The handful of people at the time who saw the potential power of health statistics were not unlike those today who are exploring new applications of modern communications and data analysis tools to help foster a precision community health approach. The revolution of the early eighteenth century took far longer than that of the early twenty-first and was far less sweeping. Yet both rested on the idea that advances in gathering information—the word *data* would not become common parlance until the age of computers was well under way—can lead to better public health.

Lemuel Shattuck was among the first to see the possibilities and was also among the most prominent and effective sanitary reformers. A bookseller from Concord, Massachusetts, Shattuck understood how statistics could demonstrate the extent of health problems and how that could generate the political interest needed to solve them. Shattuck helped found the American Statistical Association and developed a system for collecting vital statistics that would become a model for nearly a dozen states. He also developed procedures that would revolutionize the national census.[14]

Shattuck's lasting impact on public health came through his work on the 1850 *Report of the Sanitary Commission of Massachusetts*.[15] The report included fifty recommendations, built on statistical evidence, for the organization of both state and local public health agencies, including the infrastructure for collecting public health information. Most of the recommendations would eventually become standard components of American public health practice, leading Charles-Edward Amory Winslow, a bacteriologist and seminal figure in public health, to call Shattuck's *Report* "the most outstanding single 'Book of Prophesy' in the history of public health."[16]

Shattuck placed great emphasis in his report on the need to collect detailed statistical information on the causes of morbidity and mortality. In that, he was the most modern of men, a progenitor of today's data-crunchers and analysts. He was not, however, immune from the biases of his time. Most upper-class Americans, Shattuck included, knew well the health problems of the poor but simply assumed their deplorable living conditions and lack of basic hygiene reflected a parallel lack of moral fiber.

Shattuck offers something of a conundrum. He was prescient in his appreciation of the use of quantitative information, yet he was either unable or unwilling to see how that information might call some of his basic principles into question. Nevertheless, Shattuck's insights are part of the foundation of government-led efforts to improve public health and to do so on the basis, at least in part, of rigorous evidence.

The subtle advances pioneered by Shattuck would take decades to come to fruition. The more dramatic changes, on the other hand, came about in weeks or months. A new threat was working its way across Europe.

Cholera was a disease perfectly suited to the conditions found in abundance in every American city of the early nineteenth century. The disease, gruesome in its symptoms and highly fatal when left untreated, spreads by contact with an intestinal bacterium that thrives in contaminated food and water. With their limited supplies of clean water, the crowded cities that were the product of the Industrial Revolution made perfect breeding grounds, and three successive cholera pandemics swept across the globe between 1817 and 1860.

The second of those pandemics began in India in the late 1820s and spread quickly westward across central Asia. Tsar Nicholas I called out the army to check its progression; not only did that fail, it also led to riots in St. Petersburg, Sevastopol, and elsewhere. American newspapers reported exhaustively on the coming storm. In fact, no other disease, not even smallpox or yellow fever, generated as many headlines. By the time cholera reached London in late 1831, the fear of a cholera epidemic striking an American city was at a fever pitch. When word reached upstate New York that the disease had been detected in Quebec and Montreal, people began to flee their homes.[17]

Cholera struck New York in the summer of 1832 and killed some three thousand, mostly poor, residents. It spread westward for the next two years, following rivers and stagecoach routes, skipping some towns entirely while devastating others. The pattern was always the same: those who could flee in advance of the disease did so, and many of those forced to remain who contracted cholera died.[18] Among the settlements that faced the disease was a fur-trading outpost on Lake Michigan, perfectly situated between the lake and the subcontinental divide that separated the Great Lakes and the Atlantic Ocean to the east from the Mississippi River and the Gulf of Mexico to the west. Its name may have been derived from a Potawatomi word for *strong*: Chicago.

Chicago

The first plan of the town of Chicago was laid out in 1830. None of the streets on the map, most named for former US presidents, existed, and whatever crude tracks there were disappeared into a swampy morass after each heavy rain. All the muck did not slow down the speculators drawn by plans for a canal that would connect Lake Michigan to the Illinois River and then the Mississippi and eventually the Gulf of Mexico. A boom was under way, built on visions of a new city that would be the gateway to the untapped riches of the Northwest.

There were numerous obstacles to overcome before that shining city could be built. By 1854, when a cholera outbreak killed 6 percent of Chicago's roughly thirty thousand inhabitants, the city was rapidly developing a reputation as one of the unhealthiest cities in the country. Residents were using the Chicago River as a sewer because the city had no functional alternative. The river flowed into Lake Michigan, which was one of the main sources of drinking water, the other being shallow wells, which were hardly any cleaner.[19]

About the same time, efforts to understand a cholera outbreak near London led to one of the earliest uses of data in public health. A sudden and severe outbreak of cholera hit Soho, then a suburb of London. More than 127 people died in three days. Dr. John Snow, who lived nearby, happened to have a particular interest in the disease. He believed it was spread by contaminated water: most homes and businesses dumped untreated sewage and animal waste directly into the River Thames. This placed Snow in opposition to the prevailing scientific wisdom of the day, which blamed miasma—"bad air"—for making people ill. The Soho outbreak was a chance for Snow to prove his theory correct.

Snow visited each residence in the neighborhood and collected and analyzed health data related to the outbreak. The majority of Soho's cholera cases were clustered around a public water pump on nearby Broad Street. Snow used a geographic grid to chart deaths from the outbreak and investigated each case to determine access to the pump water. The proof was incontrovertible: customers of a coffee shop that used water from the pump became ill; inmates at a nearby workhouse that had its own well did not.

Dirty water from that pump, not bad air, had caused the cholera outbreak. Snow convinced town officials to remove the handle from the pump; the outbreak was over within days. It would be a tidy story if it ended there, with widespread acceptance of an elegant bit of scientific investigation, but then, as now, popular ideas did not change overnight.

Larger efforts to clean up water supplies in and around London lagged, and cholera continued to be a scourge until Robert Koch isolated the cholera bacterium in 1883 and water sanitation efforts became widespread. Still, Snow's work, alongside Lemuel Shattuck's, laid the foundation for modern epidemiology, and for precision community health.

Chicago was ahead of the curve when it came to sanitation, even if the decision was not based on any particular insight into how diseases spread. In 1855, the city council asked an engineer who had helped build water systems for Boston, Ellis Sylvester Chesbrough, to devise a sewage solution. No American city at the time had one. In the first of several remarkable feats of engineering aimed squarely at improving public health in Chicago, Chesbrough proposed creating an underground sewer system. Without a germ-based theory of disease, but with ample experience with foul-smelling water running from taps, Chesbrough had the idea to bring in enough clean water from the lake to dilute the sewage pouring into the river. The plan made perfect sense except for the fact that Chicago is mostly flat. Gravity would not drain sewage into the Chicago River. The solution was simultaneously simple and wildly ambitious: raise the city. Workers laid drains at street level and then covered them with several feet of soil. New roads and sidewalks were laid on top.[20]

That meant that homes, shops, and offices were now some six feet underground, so they would have to be raised as well. In 1858, the engineers used hundreds of jack screws to raise a four-story, 750-ton brick structure at the northeast corner of Randolph and Dearborn Streets to the new grade. More than fifty buildings were raised in similar fashion that year. By 1860, the engineers—including George Pullman, later of railroad fame—in one go, raised an entire masonry row of shops and offices taking up almost one acre and weighing thirty-five thousand tons. Crowds gathered to watch, but businesses did not even close their doors as they inched upward. By one account, when workers raised the

Tremont Hotel, the largest in the city, by eight feet, it went so smoothly that the guests, who were never asked to leave, were unaware that anything out of the ordinary was going on.[21] It is hard to believe.

Older wooden buildings were not raised; they were simply put on rollers and trundled off to the outskirts of town. All those wooden structures would prove to be problematic a few years later. Meanwhile, the new sewers improved the daily lives of Chicagoans. The sewer system, or the Chesbrough sewers, as it was known, was the first comprehensive sewer system in the United States. But the sewage still ended up in Lake Michigan, so Chesbrough also oversaw the digging of a tunnel under the lake to a spot two miles offshore that would be the main intake point for the city's water supply. Topped by a caisson and sluice gates, the tunnel was the foundation of a system that continues to supply water to a city that now is home to nearly three million people. Chesbrough's works are on the National Register of Historic Places and have been designated a Historic Civil Engineering Landmark by the American Society of Civil Engineers.[22]

With cleaner water now available in much of the city, the immediate threat of cholera began to fade. The Civil War created an urgent need for industrial development, and Chicago's manpower, transportation, and resources were perfectly placed to take advantage of the stimulus. The city boomed once again as it became a hub for grain, lumber, meatpacking, and manufacturing during the war, and its population grew fivefold. When the war ended, Chicago was a bustling, energetic city, the Gem of the Prairie, as its boosters liked to say. Chicago's future was bright.

A Hot Time in the Old Town

The summer of 1871 was hot and dry. The onset of fall brought little relief, and parched trees dropped their leaves in heaps on the streets. Outside of a few well-to-do neighborhoods along the lakeshore, Chicago was built almost entirely of wood. Most houses were made of wood, as were the barns that accompanied nearly every house and that families filled with hay for their cows or goats or flocks of chickens. The sidewalks were wood—and unfortunately raised off the ground, so they would almost act as chimneys. Wooden fences were everywhere, as were warehouses lined with wooden shelves, rail-yards full of wooden boxcars, a harbor crammed with wooden ships. Chicago had also become a center of woodworking industries, so furniture factories abounded, along with lumber mills and carriage works. Not only did that mean stores of wood scattered about the city, it meant coal to run the steam engines that powered the machinery, all of which spewed out huge quantities of sawdust. The very air itself, it seemed, might catch fire. All that was needed was a spark.

The fire that would consume much of Chicago began on the west side of town, at 137 De Koven Street. The O'Leary family lived there, along with five cows, a calf, and a horse. Mrs. O'Leary's cow may indeed have kicked over a lantern, but we'll never know for sure. But it is beyond dispute that the fire spread quickly from De Koven Street toward the central business district, fed by a strong southwest wind that only grew more persistent as the night wore on.[23]

Chicago was not utterly unprepared for a fire. The city took great pride in the waterworks building and its attendant water tower situated on the lakeshore at the foot of Chicago Avenue, built of stone and supposedly fireproof. But a timber about twelve feet long came sailing in on the wind like a flaming arrow and landed on a cornice of the waterworks, where the wood framing beneath the slate roof quickly caught fire and spread to the floors and ceilings. The heart of the city's defense against fire was gone in less than an hour. Firefighters, who had continued to battle the flames despite intense heat, low water pressure, and lack of equipment, were now helpless. The fire would burn for a day and half, consuming the most densely populated stretch of the city, block by block. By the time it burned itself out, the Great Chicago

Fire had destroyed two thousand acres and left one-third of the city's residents homeless.[24]

The death toll from the fire will never be known for certain, but it may have been as high as three hundred. Still, it could have been far worse, and without doubt, disease and other hardships of urban life in rapidly industrializing America claimed far more lives and would continue to do so for generations. Yet for sheer drama, few events of nineteenth-century American history, outside of the Civil War, can match the Great Chicago Fire. For obvious reasons, the fire defined the future of the city in nearly every regard, including its approach to public health.

The immediate impact was nearly catastrophic because the blaze leveled much of the city's medical infrastructure. Among the losses were Rush Medical College—the first medical school in the city—and six hospitals, as well as drugstores, medical offices, and libraries. The Woman's Medical College, which had opened its doors only the previous year, was also destroyed.

A combination of volunteers and officials created the Chicago Relief and Aid Society to house the homeless and try at least to prevent epidemic diseases. Sanitary officers conducted daily inspections of these makeshift quarters, and the city required a smallpox vaccination for anyone receiving relief. In spite of these efforts, smallpox, dormant since 1865, broke out. More than two thousand people contracted the disease following the fire, and more than one-fourth of those infected died. Children under five were particularly susceptible to the disease, making their mortality rate the worst in Chicago's history.[25]

The loss of life and property quite appropriately dominate any discussion of the fire, but it had another effect as well. In terms of public health, the fire in effect wiped the slate clean. Historian Thomas Neville Bonner called it a "salutary sweeping of the Augean stables before newer and greater projects were inaugurated."[26] That might be too rosy a picture, but it is true that Chesbrough's sewers and the tunnels into the lake survived largely intact, while many of the densely packed, run-down tenements were destroyed, providing Chicago with something of a clean slate on which to rebuild. The rebuilding began immediately; in fact, the first load of new lumber for construction arrived before the last burnt embers had cooled.

Planners, dreamers, and industrialists foresaw a new city, a vision that would culminate in the White City of the 1893 World's Colum-bian Exposition and from there a new, comprehensive plan that would move Chicago to the forefront of urban design. In the meantime, how-ever, Chicago saw another huge burst of immigration into the city and the re-creation of the crowded tenements that the fire had consumed. At the same time, business was booming, particularly the meatpacking industry, which deepened its hold on city politics. Both living and work-ing conditions deteriorated, particularly for the poor.

In 1876, the city reorganized its government and established a per-manent Department of Health to grapple with public health concerns. The man chosen to run the department was a forty-two-year-old army surgeon from Massachusetts named Oscar Coleman De Wolf. Over the next thirteen years, De Wolf would establish himself, and Chicago, as a leader in the public health movement.

De Wolf sought to clean up the meat-packers in his first weeks on the job. His first approach was to seek their cooperation, which he found analogous to making "the Jaguar . . . amenable to the influences of Chris-tianity."[27] He next called for sanitary inspectors to inspect meat at the slaughterhouses and confiscate any that was tainted. De Wolf attempted to move the slaughterhouses to the outskirts of the city and to curb their practice of dumping animal carcasses and chemicals into Lake Michigan and the Chicago River.

The idea of governments, at any level, intervening to improve working conditions or to stop industry from fouling the air or water was largely unheard of in the United States. Over the next four years, De Wolf fought the meatpacking companies in court and their representatives on the city council, to relatively little effect. But he had established a principle and a role for the Department of Health. He was more successful in improving housing by sending health inspectors to examine the tenements in which the immigrant poor and working classes lived. The inspectors would prove to be a key tool in a new government-led effort to improve public health, and this in a city that had little interest in placing any restrictions on the rights of landlords.[28]

The public interest in improving conditions in the tenements, where diphtheria, typhoid, cholera, smallpox, and yellow fever could take root, is readily apparent to modern eyes. But sanitary reformers such as De Wolf had to fight to be heard above the clanking din of laissez-faire capitalism. Gradually, however, city leaders began to understand that the poor endangered more than themselves when they crowded into filthy quarters.

By 1887, advancements in medical understanding also helped public health officials see that typhoid would continue to kill unless they stopped the flow of contaminated water into Lake Michigan. Solving that problem required a solution as dramatic as, or perhaps more dramatic than, raising the streets and the buildings for the sewer system. In one of the largest public health–related engineering projects the country had ever seen, engineers would attempt to permanently reverse the course of the Chicago River.

It was not the first time city officials had made such an audacious proposal. In 1871, a few months before the Great Fire, engineers had enlarged and deepened the Illinois and Michigan Canal in hopes that it would reduce the amount of sewage in the Chicago River, which had become unbearably foul smelling. Both the river and the canal would carry water west, away from the lake and into the Des Plaines River and eventually the Mississippi. The plan worked, but not well and not permanently. The old canal, which had been the lure that drew thousands to Chicago in the first place and helped make the city the shipping hub of the western United States, was not up to the task.

Although Louis Pasteur and Robert Koch had proven by the late 1870s that bacteria cause cholera, typhoid, diphtheria, and other illnesses, there was still no way to apply that knowledge to improving public health. Chicago needed a permanent solution immediately. The idea of buying up farmland on the outskirts of town and using city sewage to fertilize it was rejected because of cost and fear of the stench, even though the plan was based on the old idea of dilution. City officials decided instead to build a bigger, longer canal that would once and for all turn the Chicago River around.

Construction of the twenty-eight-mile Chicago Sanitary and Ship Canal would require innovative engineering and quite a lot of brute force. Construction began in the fall of 1892 and continued for nearly eight years. In that time workers moved more earth than in any project before, and even more than for the Panama Canal, which would not begin construction for another fourteen years. In fact, the array of different earthmoving technologies developed for the Sanitary and Ship Canal offered evidence that the long-imagined Panama Canal was more than a dream. Many lakefront cities are located at the mouth of a river, and many have considered reversing a river's flow, but only Chicago has found the technical and economic wherewithal to carry it out. In 1999, the canal and its system of locks was named a Civil Engineering Monument of the Millennium by the American Society of Civil Engineers.

The canal and related efforts to dilute sewage and carry it away from the city were successful, though downstream cities such as St. Louis were less than pleased with the results.[29] The Chicago River ran cleaner, and the stench diminished. But people were still getting ill, particularly from typhoid fever. In 1911, at long last abandoning dilution and acting on germ theory, Chicago began to sterilize its water by adding chlorine to the water supply at the pumping stations.

Within four years the entire supply was being treated, causing a dramatic decline in the city's typhoid fever rate—from the second highest among the twenty largest US cities in 1881 to the lowest by 1917. A few years later the city began construction of a sewage treatment plant, and throughout the middle of the twentieth century construction continued on the water and sewage treatment works that remain the fundamental infrastructure of the city, the largest such works of any city in the world.

Beyond Science and Engineering

The late nineteenth and early twentieth centuries saw huge leaps in the scientific understanding of the causes of disease as well as in the willingness and ability of local, state, and federal governments to act on that knowledge. Vaccination campaigns finally succeeded in defeating smallpox, after one last deadly outbreak in 1893. More vaccines, such as for diphtheria, would soon follow. Pasteurization of milk became routine, reporting of infectious disease more rigorous, and building codes a standard part of the construction business. All of that was vital to the development of effective public health efforts in Chicago and elsewhere around the country. But neither good science nor heroic engineering would be enough. Solving the most troubling problems of public health requires more than treating their individual physical manifestations and more even than addressing their environmental roots. An effective public health strategy also requires understanding how people live and why they make the choices that shape their futures, for good or ill.

In Chicago, it was not city government but a private citizen, Jane Addams, who took the initiative to address those questions and to take on the health needs of the working poor. Addams and Ellen Gates Starr opened Hull House, Chicago's first settlement house, in 1889 in a predominately immigrant neighborhood in the Nineteenth Ward, then called Halstead and today best known as the location of the University of Illinois at Chicago. In keeping with the settlement house movement as it had been established in Great Britain, Addams and Starr sought to confront poverty, poor housing conditions, disease, and other ills common to Chicago's poorest residents.

None of the Hull House founders had deep expertise in public health—Addams herself had studied medicine for a time—but they took on efforts to improve garbage collection and sanitation and to eliminate typhoid in their neighborhood. The women of Hull House knew their neighbors and their needs, they took both the people and the problems seriously, and they brought the tools of political activism to solving them.

Addams also founded the Visiting Nurse Association of Chicago to supply nurses to visit the working poor in their own homes. The association stationed nurses in twenty-five different districts in the city and supplied nurses for businesses. Hull House also played an important role in shaping a national conception of public health issues through its surveys of working-class labor and living conditions.

Businesses also stepped up and became active in addressing health concerns. In 1935, thousands of miles away, industrialist Henry J. Kaiser started providing health care to 6,500 workers and their families at the largest construction site in history—Grand Coulee Dam on the Columbia River in Washington State. Kaiser enlisted physician Sidney Garfield, who turned an existing run-down hospital into a state-of-the-art treatment facility and recruited a team of doctors to work in a "prepaid group practice." This prepayment was a new model for health care: companies would pay a fixed amount per day, per covered worker, up front. This would enable doctors to emphasize maintaining health and safety rather than merely treating illness and injury, and for a small additional charge workers could also receive coverage for medical problems that were not job related.

With the outbreak of World War II, Kaiser and Garfield expanded that approach to provide health care to ninety thousand workers at the Kaiser Shipyards in Richmond, California; Portland, Oregon; and Vancouver, Washington. When the war ended, the health plan opened its doors to the public, and in 1953 it took the name Kaiser Permanente.

Kaiser Permanente gradually began to explore how community health could affect personal health. About the same time, in the 1950s, the delivery of personal health-care services, primarily to low-income populations, was becoming the primary identity of public health in Chicago.

That identity was firmly in place when I arrived at the Chicago Department of Public Health. I was appointed on the heels of the department's response to the H1N1 influenza epidemic by setting up citywide clinics to offer flu vaccine to residents. The challenge Mayor Emanuel and I faced was to build on the strong foundation of Chicago's public health system but also to point the city in a new direction.

The CDPH is located in a beautiful building on South State Street, just a few blocks from Grant Park and the Buckingham Fountain. The office of the commissioner is down a long hallway on the second floor. The hall is lined with the official portraits of every health commissioner in the city's history, starting with Oscar Coleman De Wolf, resplendent in a bow tie and white goatee. Walking down that hallway for the first time was a powerful moment that I still think about. Not only was it a reminder of Chicago's long history of public health innovation, and of my obligation to honor that history; it was also a profound metaphor for my own journey.

Growing up in a tiny, war-torn country, I would never have imagined that I would be asked to run this agency for the third-largest city in the United States. It was humbling. It was scary. It was emotional on that first day and nearly every day thereafter. Part of the emotion stemmed from my understanding that my immigrant journey was a privileged one. Many other immigrants do not have the advantages that I did. When I arrived in Houston in 1997 to take up my residency in family medicine at Baylor College of Medicine, I saw the struggles of so many immigrants firsthand. Before moving to the United States, I had imagined a country of almost universal prosperity. Houston and Beirut would have almost nothing in common. So, I was taken aback at the poverty I saw, and that experience has stayed with me and profoundly shaped what I see as the mission of precision community health.

CHAPTER 2

Learning the Hard Way

Early on in the Rahm Emanuel administration, we did not even realize that some of the things we were trying would later fit the description of precision community health. Many of those early efforts taught us important lessons about the promise of this approach, its limitations, and the often fraught political process that would accompany any reform effort in Chicago.

My learning curve was steep, and it began long before I entered the Chicago mayor's office. At Ben Taub Hospital in Houston, Texas, one of the state's oldest and largest public hospitals, I treated homeless people with gangrenous feet and gang members with gunshot wounds. I also trained in a community health center serving mostly Mexican immigrants who struggled to make a decent living. I learned about homelessness by providing clinical services to people living in shelters, under bridges, in cars, and on the streets. Day in and day out, I saw what poverty, violence, and lack of housing does to people.

I also had an opportunity to work at Memorial Hermann-Texas Medical Center. It is basically around the corner from Ben Taub Hospital, but they are entirely different places. The lobby of Memorial looks like an elegant hotel. People come from around the world for treatment there, and the quality of care is second to none. I was grateful for the opportunity to train with some of the best doctors and in some of the best facilities anywhere. But the inequity was too striking for me to ignore.

As someone new to the United States, it was not what I expected. The experience was frankly not all that different from my medical training in Lebanon. The civil war had ended by the time I entered medical school, but the scars remained. The physical and, perhaps more telling, the mental trauma of war and displacement touched the lives of just about everyone in the country. The effects, however, were not distributed evenly. The training hospital at the American University of Beirut was, and remains, a world-class facility, attracting wealthy people from across the region, just as Memorial does in Houston. At the other end of the spectrum were the health clinics in the Palestinian refugee camps, where we were lucky to have even the most basic supplies. In Lebanon's many remote mountain villages, there was little health care, if any at all.

Consider the plight of Raheema, for example. She was fifty years old when I met her in Lebanon while I was in medical school. She was a member of the Druze community, one of the seventeen different religious sects in Lebanon. The Druze community is a wonderful, tightly connected small community living mostly in Lebanon and Syria. Raheema lived in one of the remote villages in the mountains of Lebanon. She walked to my clinic dressed in a beautiful long black robe with a white veil covering her head and part of her face. Raheema didn't have a regular doctor. In fact, she had never seen a doctor before. She had never had insurance. She had never had preventive care. She had no formal education.

Raheema walked in complaining of abdominal pain. It turned out she had a large pelvic mass and was diagnosed with metastatic cancer. The only reason she came to the clinic was that she could barely walk. She was apprehensive. She was confused.

Raheema did not choose to wait until her cancer had metastasized before seeking medical care. She was born and raised in a community that didn't prioritize access to care. Had the health-care system in Lebanon been built to support prevention, she could have discovered her cancer long before it was too late.

I discovered that there were people just like Raheema living in places such as Houston and Chicago. The surprising level of inequity in access to health care in the United States has stuck with me since those early days in Houston. It only deepened when I took on the role of medical director of Crusader Community Health, a community health center network in Rockford, Illinois, about ninety miles northwest of Chicago. There I learned about migrant communities, public housing, and HIV/AIDS, along with the brutal effects of poverty.

In 2005, I moved to Chicago and joined Heartland Alliance for Human Needs & Human Rights. I worked with immigrants and refugees on the North Side and ran a network of primary care and mental health clinics. I also worked with many of the Heartland Alliance global health teams, such as those working on HIV prevention among men who have sex with men in Nigeria, on sexual and gender-based violence in Sulaymaniyah, Iraq, and on torture and trauma treatment in Momostenango, Guatemala.

I visited some of those sites and learned from the Heartland Alliance staff. Most important, I learned from the participants in these programs. The takeaway lesson was clear: human rights and human potential cannot be separated from health. And health cannot be separated from housing or economic security or legal protections. These issues are inherently intertwined and therefore must be addressed together.

I will forever be grateful for all that I learned from people I met during my tenure at Crusader Community Health and at Heartland Alliance. The leaders in both organizations gave me the opportunity to serve and to launch my career in the United States. Gordon Eggers, Heidi Nelson, Sid Mohn: thank you.

And then fall 2009 came along. Dr. Terry Mason stepped down as health commissioner for the City of Chicago. I had never thought I would be interested in working for the government, let alone local government. But Greg Harris, one of my favorite state representatives ever, and now majority leader in the Illinois House of Representatives, encouraged me to seriously consider public service and to apply for the job. So I did. Two weeks later, Mayor Richard M. Daley asked me to become head of the Chicago Department of Public Health (CDPH).

The city's primary care and mental health care clinics were poorly managed and inefficient, and they were a source of regular complaints from city residents. Since I was then running a network of Federally Qualified Health Centers—a designation that meant we offered comprehensive services and were able to receive reimbursement from the federal government through Medicare and Medicaid—Mayor Daley saw me as someone who could turn the clinics around.

My first meeting with the mayor was intimidating; he was, of course, a Chicago legend, the son of a mayor who had served for more than twenty years and who had himself served for twenty years. He was renowned for a willingness to innovate while also being the embodiment of a gruff, big-city machine politician. What struck me in that first conversation with him was his interest in a clinic operator to run the health department. He knew that tens of thousands of Chicagoans depended on this clinic network for health care. His view of my role was mostly focused on the body and the mind. My focus was body, mind, and community. I had a much bigger agenda at heart. But I was hired for my clinical operations experience—not my vision of public health.

Even if improving the clinics was the focus, there was much else to do. Mayor Daley expected me to keep the traditional roles of the CDPH—restaurant inspections, epidemiological tracking, and so on. I did so, but I also wanted to find new ways to address health care for poor communities and bolster other systems that affect health. When I accepted the position, things had been the same for a long time. That was my first hard lesson in the realities of big-city public health: good ideas are not enough, because change does not come easy.

My goal was to transform the policies, the systems, and the environments that create health in a community. I am not sure that was what Mayor Daley or his senior advisors wanted me to focus on, save for Deputy Chief of Staff Bina Patel, who was an advocate for public health transformation in the administration and my ally in pushing a reform agenda. Daley was an effective mayor. I enjoyed getting to know him as a person and getting to know his wonderful wife, Maggie. Public health, though, was not one of his top priorities. I would not call him a public health mayor. Yes, he wanted to solve the problem of the clinics; they were costing a lot of money and providing less than adequate care. But he didn't want to take on the political battle that would be required to fix the system. This wasn't simply a matter of better management. We had to consider whether it would be best to take the city out of the business of managing clinics altogether and instead partner with nonprofits to improve care. Mayor Daley was not willing to make those tough decisions.

The reason for that unwillingness became clear in the fall of 2010, less than a year after I was hired at the CDPH, when Mayor Daley announced that he would not run for a seventh term in office. His decision not to run came as a shock—for years he had been known as "mayor for life." By the time he left office, he had served as mayor for twenty-two years, longer even than his father, the equally legendary Richard J. Daley. His departure would leave an enormous political vacuum.

I had a moment of regret for accepting the job of commissioner. I joined the department and the city government to make an impact, and it was not clear to me that I had done so. I was thinking about resigning and moving back to the private sector when I heard that Rahm Emanuel had announced that he would run for mayor. His reputation as President

Barack Obama's chief of staff was well known—brilliant, aggressive, with a habit of spewing profanity and, as they said, "breaking a lot of china." I had never met him, and I had no idea what his approach to public health might be. But I knew he was likely going to win.

President Obama had just pushed the Affordable Care Act (ACA), and Emanuel had been instrumental in making that happen. That was reason enough to be optimistic about the approach he might take as mayor. The ACA, in my mind, was desperately needed for the people in this country, both to increase access to care and coverage and to reshape how health care is practiced. We began to have a broad public debate about whether health care is a human right or a privilege. That moment in the Barack Obama–John McCain debate when the two presidential candidates expressed totally opposing views on this is still vivid in my mind—Senator Obama said health care was a right of every American, while Senator McCain said it was the responsibility of individuals to obtain insurance themselves, glossing over the often insurmountable obstacles many people face in getting insurance through private markets.

It was clear to me that as mayor, Rahm Emanuel would take the idea of body, mind, community seriously. After a year on the job in the Daley administration, I was coming to the conclusion that simply making the public health clinics more efficient was not going to address underlying problems that stemmed from long histories of discrimination and neglect. We were treating a symptom while neglecting the underlying causes of the problem. We needed something more dramatic, but we had no guidebook, no broadly accepted models to draw on. I was ever more convinced that we could make great strides if we could leverage data and information in new ways while at the same time keeping our focus on improving the lives of Chicagoans. Mayor Daley, at the end of a long career, was not interested in taking on something that everyone knew would be risky and controversial. Rahm Emanuel, on the other hand, seemed to be poised for a change agenda. I wanted to be part of that journey. I had not seen myself as a politician, but I was about to get an education in Chicago's rough-and-tumble brand of politics. And I still have the scars to prove it.

City of Neighborhoods

When I took over at the CDPH, I had not lived in the city long enough to learn the nuances of such a complicated place, with a long history of both triumph and tribulation. I knew enough about Chicago to understand that the challenge for the city, and for many other places around the country, is the disparity in health outcomes for different racial and ethnic groups. What took longer for me to really appreciate was that the roots of that disparity run deep. In Chicago, they stem in part from the way the city grew, particularly during the period of rapid expansion of the city's population in the first half of the twentieth century.

Chicago calls itself the City of Neighborhoods. Of course, every city has them, but in Chicago they are an especially important part of how residents see themselves.[1] City government recognizes seventy-seven neighborhoods—officially called community areas—and they serve as the basis for a variety of urban planning initiatives on both the local and regional levels. The Social Science Research Committee at the University of Chicago defined seventy-five community areas during the late 1920s. At the time, these areas corresponded roughly to neighborhoods or interrelated neighborhoods within the city. While residents may use different names for more compact parts of the community areas, the map has been remarkably stable, with only two additions in nearly a century.

More telling than the boundaries, however, has been the stability—for good and ill—of the neighborhoods and their makeup. Many Chicagoans see themselves as deeply connected to their neighborhoods, sometimes more so than to the city as a whole. They are from Uptown or Back of the Yards or Calumet Heights first, or even from the parish in which they live, sometimes even if they are not Catholic. That has shaped the city for generations and continues to contribute to its abiding strength and diversity. Chicago is a more vibrant, livable place because of the deep roots people have here.

But there is a far less pleasant underside to this story, one that plays out in terms of economic opportunity and public health. Chicago's neighborhoods reflect a legacy of segregation that dates back to the Great Migration, the movement of some seven million African Americans out of the rural South to cities such as Chicago, Detroit, Pittsburgh, and elsewhere between 1916 and 1970. About five hundred thousand African Americans relocated to Chicago in this era, and the percentage of city residents who were African American grew from 2 percent to 33 percent by 1970.

Chicago offered economic opportunities to African Americans that were denied to them in the South, especially after World War I began and cut off the flow of European immigrants. Factories in need of labor opened their gates to African American men, and while women were still largely restricted to cleaning houses and other domestic jobs, these still paid better than what was available in the South. The city offered a haven from the worst depredations of the Jim Crow era, but African Americans received far from equal treatment.

According to the journalist and author Isabel Wilkerson, who chronicled the Great Migration in *The Warmth of Other Suns*, many of those arriving in Chicago were confined to an area on the South Side that is today called Bronzeville but was also known as the Black Belt or North Mississippi. It was a long and narrow stretch of the city, about ten square miles, but it became home to nearly all African Americans arriving from the South. They were squeezed between Jewish neighborhoods along the lake to the east and Irish neighborhoods to the west. But people kept coming, and not just from the South. The lure of factory jobs was powerful enough that even the prospect of moving into an attic or a storeroom or someone's shed was hardly an impediment.

The new arrivals in Chicago paid the highest rents for the worst housing. From a public health perspective, this kind of discrimination has been devastating and among the hardest problems to root out. That is true not only in Chicago. As Wilkerson notes, the overcharging and underinvestment in black neighborhoods laid the foundation for economic disparities in cities across the northern United States. But Chicago's case is illustrative, and I saw the effects firsthand.

The resistance of white residents to the influx of African Americans during the Great Migration was fierce, sometimes violent, often illegal, but sadly effective in many places. African Americans looking to buy a home not only faced restrictive covenants meant to keep white neighborhoods white; they were also victims of predatory lending that could leave them broke as well as homeless. All of this seems to have occurred with the explicit backing of the federal government, which made mortgage insurance available to neighborhoods on the basis of their perceived stability. Predominantly white neighborhoods were rated A and were colored green on official maps; largely black neighborhoods were rated D, were ineligible for insurance, and were colored red. "Redlining" spread from the government to nearly all mortgage banking, with devastating effects on the quality of housing available for poorer, minority residents of the city.

Segregation has fallen in Chicago, yet the disparity remains in place. Nationwide, segregation in urban areas has declined, and a 2012 study by the Manhattan Institute for Policy Research found that Chicago had the second-largest decline in the country, after Houston. But the same study also found that Chicago remains the most racially segregated city in the country.[2]

While parts of Chicago have blossomed, poor families are often cut off from the growth. The factories that once dotted Chicago's South and

West Sides have moved overseas or to the suburbs. The schools are worse, and health care is often hard to find. Now there is a second great migration under way, this time away from the city: between 2000 and 2010, some 180,000 black residents of Chicago moved out, either to other cities—many, ironically, in the South that are now less segregated—or to the suburbs. Those who moved were usually economically secure, middle-class people; those left behind were poor, further driving the downward spiral of some neighborhoods.

When I arrived in Chicago in 2005, the depths of the problem and its consequences were apparent to anyone willing to look with an unbiased eye. As late as 2002, some academics were still debating the link between income inequality and public health,[3] but few people on the front lines could deny the evidence. Shortly after I was appointed at the CDPH, Northwestern University undertook a comprehensive study, the first to build a profile of the health of residents and resources in Chicago neighborhoods. The study looked at the prevalence of five key public health issues for the entire city: childhood obesity, breast cancer, HIV/AIDS, teen pregnancy, and motor vehicle injury and death. The Centers for Disease Control and Prevention (CDC) calls these "winnable battles" because they have large-scale impact and known, effective strategies to address them. The study also tracked assets such as parks, easy access to high-quality medical care, safe places to exercise, and stores that sell affordable healthy foods such as fresh fruits and vegetables.

The results confirmed what we were seeing nearly every day, but they were striking and disturbing nonetheless. For example, in 2009, a higher proportion of black (22.6 percent) and Hispanic/Latino (22.4 percent) Chicago high school students were overweight, compared with white students (11.8 percent). In 2008, blacks in Chicago accounted for 60 percent of the HIV diagnoses in adolescents and adults despite representing one-third of Chicago's population, and nearly all teen births occurred among black and Latina young women. The south and southwest regions of Chicago have the highest breast cancer mortality rates, but few breast health services, such as mammogram testing sites, exist for women in these areas. Rather, breast health resources are concentrated in the north and northwest regions, which also have the lowest breast cancer mortality rate.

Since then, further studies have shown how pervasive the problem is in this country. Income inequality has increased over the past four decades, and it is now so severe that the United States is more unequal, as measured by the gap in household disposable income between richest and poorest 10 percent, than any country besides Chile, Mexico, and Turkey.[4] The United States also has higher rates of infant mortality and shorter life expectancy than other wealthy nations. Those facts by themselves should shock the conscience of every American, but when you scratch beneath the surface of such global comparisons, the impact on communities and individuals is even more disturbing.

While middle-income and high-income Americans are living longer, poor Americans have seen no such improvement, and their lives in some cases may actually be shorter now than they were in the 1980s, according to a report from the National Academies of Sciences, Engineering, and Medicine.[5] The life expectancy of the wealthiest 1 percent of Americans now exceeds that of the poorest 1 percent by over ten years among men and nearly fifteen years among women. The pattern is as consistent as it is outrageous: nearly any chronic condition you look at, be it stroke, heart disease, or arthritis, is more common the further down the income scale you go.[6]

Saddest of all is the pattern we see for infant mortality, defined as the number of deaths under one year of age per 1,000 live births. In 2016, I served on a committee of the National Academies that examined the problem of health inequality. Among the findings we reported was that infant mortality was much higher in certain populations. In 2013, among non-Hispanic whites, 5.06 infants of every 1,000 live births died before their first birthday; among African Americans, that rate was double, at 11.1 per 1,000. Rates were also higher for Native American (7.61 per 1,000) and Puerto Rican (5.93 per 1,000) infants, as well as for low-income white infants in the Appalachian region, where in 2012, 7.6 infants died for every 1,000 live births.[7]

The problem is not just that people living in poorer communities are more likely to smoke, be overweight, or use drugs; they also confront unequal access to technological innovations, increased geographic segregation by income, reduced economic mobility, mass incarceration, and more expensive medical care. Low-income Americans are being left behind in so many ways, and it is entirely predictable that this undeniable fact would have a long-term impact on their health.

Our National Academies report, issued in early 2017, showed that the burdens of poor health and the benefits of good health are inequitably distributed in the United States as a result of factors that range from poverty and inadequate housing to structural racism and discrimination. The last factor is still a difficult one for academics, policy makers, scientists, elected officials, journalists, and others to face or address in a constructive fashion, despite growing evidence of its importance. For someone who was born outside the United States, this is particularly difficult to comprehend.

We need to look no further than what happened in Flint, Michigan, to see the awful power of structural racism: the ways in which societies foster racial discrimination through mutually reinforcing systems of housing, education, employment, earnings, benefits, credit, media, health care, and criminal justice.[8] In 2014, still reeling from the Great Recession, the city of Flint switched from its longtime water supplier, the Detroit Water and Sewerage Department, which got its water from Lake Huron, to the Flint River. The Flint River water was far more polluted, and using it would require restarting a long-idle treatment plant, but it would save the city money. Monthly rates in Flint were among the most expensive in the country, and yet 42 percent of residents lived below the federal poverty level. And the rates kept rising.

Flint's new plan would lower water bills, but unfortunately its water treatment program did not seem to include corrosion control, in violation of federal law. Older cities such as Flint are required to add corrosion control treatment because without it the old lead pipes disintegrate and leach lead directly into the tap water of residents.

There were warning signs almost immediately after the switch, the most worrisome of which was that a General Motors plant had to go back to using water from Detroit because the Flint River water was corroding its machinery. Flint could have switched back as well but chose not to, in the mistaken belief that the problems could be repaired. They could not be, at least not in a timely fashion. Lead levels in the water skyrocketed. Just a few months after Flint switched to the river for its water, the lead levels reached 13,200 parts per billion. The level that triggers federal action is 15 parts per billion. But neither state nor federal agencies, including the US Environmental Protection Agency, seem to have acted for months.[9]

In late 2015, a Flint pediatrician, Mona Hanna-Attisha, provided the first documentation of dangerously high lead levels in children's blood.[10] Her research, confirmed by an independent team from Virginia Tech, showed that lead contamination had nearly doubled and even tripled in children younger than five after the city's water supply was switched to the Flint River. Three years later the city returned to Great Lakes water, but people were still drinking bottled water as late as mid-2018, four years after the crisis began.

The situation in Flint was shocking but, sadly, not unexpected. It fits a long-established pattern: we are entirely too ready to tolerate pollution if the communities it affects are predominantly minority and poor. The majority of people who live close to commercial hazardous waste sites are people of color; children of color represent two-thirds of kids who live within a mile of chemical facilities. A 2012 study conducted by researchers at the Yale School of Medicine found that counties in the United States with the lowest air quality, as measured by exposure to fine particulate matter, also had higher percentages of African Americans and poor people than counties with the highest-quality air.[11]

The same pattern is all too apparent when we measure health outcomes. In our National Academies study, we found that the most promising way to promote health equity—the state in which no one's health is damaged because of their place in society—is through community-driven interventions that specifically target social factors.

Health inequity is not a problem just for those whose physical well-being is so directly and tangibly at risk. It is a societal concern with profound ethical dimensions. There may be no greater responsibility for a society than to make sure everyone has the opportunity to thrive. As Mohandas Gandhi said, "A nation's greatness is measured by how it treats its weakest members."

Even if you can set aside those concerns, there are practical and immediate consequences of health inequity. It is, for one thing, extremely expensive. For example, one analysis found that eliminating health disparities for minorities would save nearly $230 billion in direct medical care expenditures over four years. When you add indirect costs, the savings total $1.24 trillion.[12] A 2009 analysis by the Urban Institute projected that from 2009 to 2018, racial disparities in health would cost US health insurers a total of approximately $337 billion.[13]

The cost of health inequity cannot, however, be measured solely in the dollars and cents we as a nation spend on health care. We must also consider national security, business viability, and economic productivity. Young adults who have spent their entire lives without adequate health care are far less likely to be able to take on the rigors of military service. The impact of poor health on private businesses may be just as significant. More research from the Urban Institute shows that young adults with health problems who cannot find jobs in the mainstream economy are less productive and generate higher health-care costs for businesses.[14]

Most important, health equity is about making sure that everyone has the ability to thrive. All people have the right to live the life they want to live. Inequities prevent that.

I have always believed that racial and economic disparities in public health are completely unacceptable. But in Chicago, such disparities were both persistent and pernicious. Getting past them would require targeting our efforts to those most in need—public health, after all, was just one of the challenges Chicago needed to address, and the city's finances were strapped. That meant making hard choices about how best to deliver public health services, and hard choices inevitably mean navigating a course through conflicting interests, some of which, I discovered, could be irreconcilable.

Healthy Chicago

My first task as commissioner was to determine how we should focus our energy as a department. There were many options, but over and over again I was struck by how creating a supportive environment for vulnerable people could help solve so many health issues.

Take diabetes, for instance, a real problem in Chicago, as in many other big cities across the country. We knew that blacks with diabetes in Chicago had a much greater risk of needing to have a limb amputated as a result of the disease than whites—in fact, the rate would turn out to be almost double among black residents of the city.[15]

Losing a leg from diabetes isn't a given, nor are racial differences in this health outcome. We know how to prevent diabetes-related complications such as limb amputations, blindness, and kidney failure. Controlling blood sugar, blood pressure, and cholesterol can significantly reduce the risk of complications and improve quality of life.

The problem is that lifestyle changes to control diabetes (e.g., healthy eating, regular physical activity, taking medications, and regular visits to the doctor) are often a challenge, particularly in low-income minority communities where resources are limited. People with diabetes are supposed to do 150 minutes of physical activity every week and eat vegetables as a key element in their diet. Concerns about crime have driven many indoors, and food deserts make purchasing fresh produce difficult.

We needed more communities where making the healthy choice is the easy choice—that is, communities with safe places to exercise; affordable, healthy food; walkable neighborhoods with safe sidewalks and bike paths; and much more. That would require taking a much broader view of the role of the CDPH than had been the case since its founding. I spent some time learning about what other health departments were doing and discovered that the CDPH was right in the middle of the pack or maybe even further behind. Places such as New York and Los Angeles were leading the way, so I sat down with people such as Thomas Frieden, at the time head of the CDC in Atlanta, Georgia, but also the former commissioner of health for New York City—where he had put the city at the forefront of public efforts to combat chronic diseases such as diabetes[16]—and Jonathan Fielding, head of the Los Angeles County Department of Public Health, a leader in the development of evidence-based public health.[17] I also had the opportunity to spend time with Barbara Ferrer, who at the time was executive director of the Boston Public Health Commission. I had much to learn from people such as Tom, Jonathan, and Barbara. And I am forever grateful for the time they gave me and the guidance they provided.

The news was not all bad. Life expectancy—in every single neighborhood—was beginning to climb. In fact, life expectancy in Chicago grew by more than seven years between 1990 and 2010, nearly twice as fast as the national average increase. This offered some reason to believe that the city was moving in the right direction. Differences in life expectancy between non-Hispanic blacks and non-Hispanic whites decreased by 10 percent, while differences between the two groups due to perinatal conditions decreased by 50 percent. Overall, Hispanic residents had a life expectancy rate of 84.7 years, the highest rate in the city.[18]

We were beginning to piece together a plan by late 2010. The mayoral election was to be held in February 2011, but I still had no idea what to expect when Rahm was elected. Would he ask me to stay? The word was that he was coming with a big change agenda and was likely to change all the cabinet members. I wasn't sure what to expect. I did lots of research to see what happened when Obama was elected and Rahm was his chief of staff. I figured he would do the same in Chicago as mayor.

Emanuel easily won the election, and his transition team reached out to me shortly thereafter. I had several conversations with them and came away with three clear ideas: reform primary care clinics; reform mental health care; and develop a broad, comprehensive plan to make Chicago the healthiest city in the country. David Spielfogel, one of people leading the transition, really liked the first two ideas. I wanted all of them. David told me that they were interested in bringing new people to the cabinet. They had already decided who among the sitting cabinet members would leave and the couple of leaders who would remain. Then there was one cabinet member whom they could not decide whether he should stay or go. That was me.

I talked to David some more and again pitched him on my three-point plan. He came around and asked me to meet with Rahm.

When I went to the transition office to meet with Rahm, it was packed and full of energy. There were many young staffers bustling around. The contrast with my first meeting with Mayor Daley could not have been starker. I was in an office waiting for Rahm and he walked in. "Hi. I am Rahm. I hear you're Lebanese American." "I am," I replied. "Are you Christian Lebanese or Muslim Lebanese?" You might think that I would have been offended by such a blunt and personal question. In fact, I was kind of impressed, because it showed both an understanding of the Middle East and a refreshingly forthright approach. When I was growing up during the war, most people in Lebanon, unfortunately, divided the world that way, and if anything the extremism has only gotten worse since. If your family name, like mine, is found in both the Muslim and Christian communities in Lebanon, people will go through all sorts of contortions to find out on what side of the line you fall, asking where you grew up, what part of the city you live in, where you went to school, all in an effort to get an answer to the question they are really interested in but without having to come right out and ask. Rahm cut though that all.

When I told family and friends in Lebanon that I would likely be working for Rahm Emanuel, a few were concerned. There had been rumors ever since Obama's election in 2008 that Rahm had served in the Israel Defense Forces during the 1982 invasion of Lebanon—an event about which I had strong feelings. It turned out that this is not true; Rahm had a two-week stint as a civilian volunteer during the 1991 Gulf War, helping repair vehicles on a military base. In any event, it was clear from talking with him that he knew a great deal about the region, and we quickly moved to talk about the role he wanted me to play. Rahm loved all three points on my plan, particularly the idea for a comprehensive public health agenda. I really liked the guy. I knew we would have a great working relationship. I knew I had the job.

Mayor Emanuel and I wanted to establish Chicago as a leader in creating healthy communities. We quickly identified tobacco, obesity, and breast cancer disparities in Chicago as key winnable battles, while also realizing that even winnable battles depend on the underlying plan and the more challenging goals ahead. That's how we started thinking about Healthy Chicago, the city's first comprehensive public health agenda.

Healthy Chicago identified nine other priority areas in addition to tobacco, obesity, and breast cancer: HIV prevention, adolescent health, heart disease, access to health care, healthy mothers, communicable disease, healthy homes, violence prevention, and emergency preparedness. In what would prove to be the first step in a precision approach to community health in Chicago, we developed sixteen health outcome measures and set targets for each one. Some were firmly in the tradition of public health practice in the United States, such as the infant mortality rate or the number of tuberculosis cases. The infant mortality rate in Chicago was 11.5 deaths per 1,000 live births; we set a target of reducing that to 7 by 2020. There were 463 cases of tuberculosis in Chicago in 1999, and we wanted to reduce that to 100 by 2020. But some of the other measures were brand-new, such as the percentage of high school students who have experienced dating violence and the percentage of adults who have been told by a doctor that they have high blood pressure.

The targets we set in Healthy Chicago created a dashboard that would tell us if the city was getting healthier. We developed more than two hundred strategies to reach the targets. We laid out the policies, including regulatory changes and law, necessary to improve the public's health, the programs and services that we would deliver, and the education and public awareness efforts that would reinforce our proposed policies and programs.

The mayor and I saw Healthy Chicago as more than just a plan. It was a call to action. For the first time, we had a citywide plan that called on all Chicagoans—the educational institutions, philanthropy, faith-based communities, the business community, neighborhood families, and individuals—to join in to transform the health of the city.

I wanted to achieve four main things by releasing Healthy Chicago. First, I wanted to identify key public health priorities. Second, I wanted to set measurable targets that we wanted to achieve by 2020 and make those targets public. Third, I wanted to identify sets of policies, interventions, and health education strategies to help us get there and also make those public. And fourth, I wanted to find meaningful ways to engage the different stakeholders in our communities to achieve the targets.

We looked at plans other cities had developed. We looked at practices across the United States and even globally to see what was most promising. We looked at the literature to identify policies, programs, and health education strategies that we could implement in Chicago. I was just starting to understand the importance of an evidence-based approach to community health, and I had a lot to learn about predictive analytics, big data, data science, artificial intelligence, and so on, but I was sure we could do better. We could be more accountable to the people who depended on us; we could be clear about what we were going to achieve and how much progress we were making. I didn't know exactly what that would look like when we launched this effort, but I knew there were people outside the public health industry who could help us bridge the gap and push innovation in a sector that has often been too willing to rely on what has worked in the past.

Seattle, for example, was an early leader in the fight against childhood obesity, a key goal for Healthy Chicago as well. In 2003, King County, which surrounds the city, moved to get fatty, salty snacks out of vending machines in schools and replace them with healthier alternatives such as yogurt and trail mixes. Obesity and poor nutrition are also serious problems in Chicago. More than half of Chicago adults and one-third of youth are overweight or obese, meaning they are at increased risk for serious, costly health problems such as heart disease and diabetes. Furthermore, nearly half of Chicagoans eat fewer than three servings of fruits and vegetables per day. It's often difficult for Chicagoans to eat nutritious food outside the home because there are few healthy options—especially in vending machines.

So we developed a tool kit to provide healthy vending guidelines and examples of how people in Chicago could start making improvements at their workplaces. Our goal was to improve choices not just in schools but also in hospitals, government offices, and private businesses of all kinds.

Healthy vending is now big business. You can even get salad from a vending machine, thanks to a Chicago-based company called Farmer's Fridge. Since 2013, nearly two hundred salad-vending machines have popped up throughout Chicago and Milwaukee, Wisconsin, in airports, universities, hospitals, and shopping areas. The company raised thirty million dollars in venture capital in 2018 and plans to add four hundred to five hundred more "fridges" in other midwestern cities such as Detroit, Indianapolis, Cincinnati, and St. Louis. Another company, HUMAN Healthy Vending (the acronym stands for Helping Unite Mankind and Nutrition), sells vending machine franchises across the country, with healthy snacks that franchise owners can customize to local markets and tastes.

That was all good news, and I will address other elements of the Healthy Chicago plan in subsequent chapters, particularly the new tools we used to meet our goals for the city. But there were important lessons to learn first. The biggest learning experience of all was our effort to reform the city's primary care and mental health care programs. As I saw it at the time, the priority was to make sure that we were investing public dollars in the right way and in the right places.

It was time to take on the clinics that Mayor Daley had charged me with reforming when I was first appointed commissioner. But now I had the leeway to make major changes, not just tweaks in management. So we began the controversial process of transitioning the clinics out of public hands to private, not-for-profit Federally Qualified Health Centers. Nationwide, Federally Qualified Health Centers now serve more than twenty-five million people.[19]

In general, these clinics are a great asset in communities across the country and often offer better care than our city-run clinics could provide. Nonetheless, *privatization* is an ugly word in the public health community, and with good reason. It often means increased profits for companies and fewer services for many people, especially the poor. That was the opposite of what we wanted for Chicago. Our goal was simple: better care at a lower cost.

That is exactly what we saw. Transitioning the public clinics to not-for-profit health centers resulted in expanded access to care, new service options, and an improved patient experience across the city. Access to care continues to expand in all seven communities that had been served by the public clinics. Following the transition period in 2012, our partners saw an increase of 32 percent in patient visits in the first half of 2013, and a 69 percent increase in the second half of 2013, compared with the first six months of 2012. And all this saved taxpayers twelve million dollars annually.

Recognizing that innovation is required to best serve residents, many of the new clinics expanded services on-site, with a special focus on preventive services. Through a partnership between Aunt Martha's, which operates seventeen community health centers, and Roseland Community Hospital on the South Side, women are efficiently connected to both primary care and breast cancer screening in the convenience of their own neighborhood. Additionally, the various partners now provide oral health services, urgent care clinics, occupational therapy, weight management and exercise classes, diabetes education, podiatry services, and more.

We found other ways to collaborate with our not-for-profit partners as well. In our effort to address diabetes, for example, the CDPH began working with organizations such as the Chicago Center for Diabetes Translation Research (CCDTR) at the University of Chicago. Together, we identified community hot spots of preventable diabetes-related hospitalizations, informing us where to concentrate disease prevention programs.

The South Side Diabetes Project, supported by the CCDTR, the Merck Foundation's Alliance to Reduce Disparities in Diabetes, and the National Institutes of Health, was another collaborative effort to improve primary care and to lower costs. The project sought to reduce diabetes disparities by involving multiple stakeholders—the CDPH, clinicians and health systems, patients, advocacy organizations, the Chicago Park District, businesses, and community organizations.

For example, the South Side Diabetes Project provides the Food Rx program (prescription-like lists of healthy foods, with vouchers redeemable at participating Walgreens stores and a local farmer's market) and "exercise prescriptions" for six months of free access to exercise facilities at city parks. The project conducts weekly tours of the low-cost grocer Save-A-Lot to help residents learn how to shop for healthy foods on limited budgets. The South Side Diabetes Project provides a real-world example of how to leverage local assets to improve community health and reduce disparities.

The Mental Health Challenge

While the shift to private providers for primary health care in Chicago was controversial, it was hardly rancorous. A change in the city's approach to behavioral health, however, was a much different and far more troubling story.

I had long been concerned about the challenge of mental health, particularly among children. I knew the devastating impact trauma can have on children because I had lived it. During the war in Lebanon, my elementary school was open only when it was safe for us to get there. And when we could go, I worried constantly that my parents would not make it home safely after they dropped my sister and me off. If we were home and my parents went out, my sister, Cynthia, got in the habit of counting the tiles on our patio, seeing how many she could count before they returned. It was a way to keep the fear and anxiety at bay.

These things happen to everyone, globally. Children in Chicago may not live in a war zone, but they still have to worry about violence, both in school and at home. And the impact may be lifelong.

From 1995 to 1997, the CDC and Kaiser Permanente conducted a study of trauma in childhood. The study revealed that the greater the number of adverse childhood experiences—such as abuse and household dysfunction—the more likely and the greater the burden of chronic illnesses, including diabetes, cancer, heart disease, chronic lung disease, substance use disorder, and mental health problems.[20] The results of this study have since been validated in more than 1,500 peer-reviewed studies.

So, there is a graded dose-response relationship between trauma and poor health throughout one's life. This is toxic stress, and the impact is as severe as for any other deadly toxin in the environment. Addressing that problem is a key to any long-term approach to community mental health.

Chicago was one of a few large cities that ran its own mental health centers. While the CDPH saw itself as a mental health care "provider of last resort," there are real advantages to having the public sector provide care. For one thing, that arrangement offers continuity of care for people who need services the most. Perhaps more significant is the intangible benefit that comes with seeing mental health care as a civic responsibility.

But the downsides are significant as well. Public mental health care can be expensive and inefficient, and the quality of the services is not always on par with what is available through private providers. As a result, places such as New York, Los Angeles, Houston, and most other big cities have shifted to a model in which nonprofit agencies provide mental health services under contract and Medicaid pays the bills. In fact, a 2013 analysis by the National Association of County and City Health Officials found that just 10 percent of local health departments provide behavioral or mental health services either directly or through contracts. Even more telling, big-city health departments are often understaffed, and this is a particularly acute problem for mental health services. Many health departments employ no full-time behavioral health professionals.[21]

In Chicago we did far better than that, but we still did not have enough professionals on staff to meet our needs. Between 2006 and 2012 the number of full-time equivalent psychiatrists employed by the city decreased by half, and we had a hard time filling vacancies even with aggressive advertising and a promise to increase the salary. But given the state of the budget, the sad fact was that we were simply not in a position to match the salary even for other public positions elsewhere in the Great Lakes, to say nothing of what a qualified psychiatrist would be paid in private practice.

During the recession that began in late 2007, state health-care budgets were under severe strain across the country. Illinois was hardly immune, but the impact was particularly severe for mental health care. From 2009 to 2012, the state, under Governor Pat Quinn, cut mental health spending by $187 million, the fourth-largest percentage decrease among all states during those years. Thousands of Chicagoans were at risk of losing psychiatric care and other vital services.

With continued cuts in funding and ongoing hiring challenges, the number of patients seen at the CDPH began to drop. By 2012, CDPH mental health centers were operating at an average capacity of just 61 percent for therapy. When the Affordable Care Act (ACA) was signed in 2010, it included a provision to expand Medicaid and held the promise of significantly increasing the number of Americans covered by health insurance. Twenty-seven states, including Illinois, opted in to the plan, which means the federal government—rather than states—would pay for treatment of newly qualified low-income people. In Illinois, we expected that just over 277,000 persons with serious mental illness or serious psychological distress would become newly eligible for coverage under the ACA—120,000 through the expanded Medicaid program and the remainder through the Illinois Health Insurance Marketplace.

While coverage information specific to persons with mental health problems is not available, in Chicago nearly 300,000 residents gained coverage once the Marketplace and Medicaid expansion began, in January 2014. Nearly 75 percent of these newly enrolled individuals became insured under the expanded Medicaid program.

We decided that the best way to spend a shrinking budget for mental health was to focus on the uninsured population, recognizing that this population has fewer options than individuals with private or public coverage. We also wanted to help the newly insured transition away from city-run clinics to private, not-for-profit providers. At the same time, we needed to make the way we provided care more efficient, so we took the controversial step of consolidating our city's twelve mental health clinics into six, at the same time increasing funding to strengthen the overall mental health infrastructure.

At the time, the CDPH committed to retaining the capacity to serve mostly uninsured and Medicaid recipients. Even though we consolidated our mental health clinics from twelve to six, the majority of clinical staff and all psychiatrists were retained.

I knew that two key groups would initially be upset by the plan to consolidate the clinics. The first obviously would be communities that had been served by the clinics that were consolidating. The second was the labor unions that represented the staffs of the public clinics. We engaged in a lot of discussions in the communities that were impacted by the plan. Many were able to see the value of the reform. A number of community-based organizations supported the plan and were on record as supporting efforts to work with the not-for-profit sector. But others remained opposed. On the labor union side, things were more controversial. In their fierce advocacy for living wages and good working conditions, labor unions have been vital to improving public health across the country. Unions have always been strong allies for public health departments, but they also have an obligation to represent their members, in this case the people whose jobs at Chicago's public mental health clinics were at risk. I was hopeful that we would get to a point where we were working closely with the labor unions to both improve mental health services and preserve jobs.

It didn't work out that way. The result ended up being a long, bruising political battle. People protested in the streets. The unions were effective at mobilizing public opinion, even if their tactics were at times questionable, such as busing people with mental illnesses to take part in street protests against the plan to reform the mental health system in Chicago.

In December 2011, shortly after we announced the plan, one protestor came to city hall dressed as Santa Claus, wearing a Mayor Emanuel mask, and carrying a sign that read, "The Grinch who stole clinics." And the furor did not die down. In June 2012, six people were arrested during a demonstration at my office; one activist called me a "butcher" and demanded my resignation. I have always been and continue to be a cheerleader for the role labor unions play in improving community health. They will always be key public health allies, but I still have the scars from that fight.

Some positive changes have come out of the reform: the remaining clinics ended up being better staffed and providing better services, and more money is going to local agencies to fill the gaps, though it is not just government employees who are doing the work.

When we consolidated the mental health centers in mid-2012, we simultaneously awarded funding to seven agency partners to increase community capacity for psychiatry services for uninsured persons. We added an eighth partner, and we continued to provide funding and made sure every single patient was connected to care. Anyone who was unhappy with the services at the private clinics could switch back to the city-run services. With the capacity created by the consolidation, by the end of 2012 the CDPH was serving new patients, all of whom were either uninsured or receiving Medicaid.

The system is still far from perfect, but it is certainly better in important ways. This experience in mental health care reform revealed the limits of consensus and coalition and also the importance of having the public firmly on your side.

Good ideas are not enough; you need to be able to put them to work. Sometimes, as we will see in the next chapter, that means a painstaking process of building grassroots support. At other times, as with the primary care clinics in Chicago, a thoughtful, well-executed transition to not-for-profit providers is the best way to go.

The experience also reinforced the importance of paying close attention to public opinion. Public opinion was on the side of keeping the status quo. The new mayor of Chicago, Lori Lightfoot, said during her campaign that she would reopen some of the mental health clinics. Since winning the election, however, she has taken a more cautious approach. According to her advisors, the new mayor hopes to increase access to mental health treatment for city residents with funds from a new real estate transfer tax, and she will increase seed funding for private centers and try to boost Medicaid reimbursement.

All this points to the complexity of the issue, both in Chicago and nationwide. The fact is, and as no doubt Mayor Lightfoot is learning, there is almost no way a public mental health care system could have delivered the care needed with the limited resources we had. It was not even close, which is why we took the steps we did. We would have had to pour in huge amounts of money that we simply did not have. The same problem, I am afraid, could well undermine plans to expand Medicare to everyone.

Violence and Public Health

Perhaps the most important lesson I took from the mental health clinic controversy was that there were no easy answers, and whatever course we chose would have real impacts on the lives of people across the city. That was brought home even more forcefully as we began to tackle the challenge of preventing gun violence, an issue that has moved to the center of public debate in Chicago over the past several years. One innovative approach to the problem gets to the heart of precision community health—both its potential and its limits.

The idea, based on work by University of Illinois at Chicago epidemiologist Gary Slutkin, was to treat violence the way we would treat an outbreak of an infectious disease. Slutkin, who has worked on tuberculosis and cholera epidemics around the world, sees violence in the same light: it's contagious, and if you don't isolate it, it can spread rapidly and with devastating effects.

Slutkin argues that the key steps are to detect ongoing and new epidemics; determine who is most likely to spread the disease and then reduce their likelihood of developing it and subsequently transmitting it; and change the underlying conditions that help spread the infection.[22]

In the late 1990s, Slutkin developed an approach, first called CeaseFire and now known as Cure Violence, that uses these same principles to prevent epidemic violence. The first pilot program took place in the Chicago neighborhood of West Garfield Park in 2000. It is, Slutkin says, both a science and community/street-based intervention, and it also embodies many of the principles that we now see in precision community health. It begins by analyzing clusters of violence and how the violence spreads and then attempts to interrupt the "transmission" of violence, ultimately changing the underlying norms that promote it. Workers are trained as "violence interrupters, outreach behavior change agents, and community coordinators" and use strategies similar to health workers looking for the first cases of bird flu or SARS.[23] The interrupters include former gang members and other ex-offenders who use their connections and street credibility to defuse potential violence before it boils over.

Cure Violence had made some important strides and helped change the way we think about the problem of urban violence. I had met Gary through public health circles years ago, and I was excited to bring his perspective into the health department.

The program used the precision community health approach of targeting specific communities with tools designed to meet their unique needs. But it also had elements of traditional public health work, investing now for results that might not be visible for some time. Unfortunately, when it comes to violence, most communities are not willing to wait, and with good reason. They need results now, and we did not provide them. While the approach has worked in some neighborhoods in Baltimore and New York, in Chicago the efforts did not gel with the police department and never felt fully integrated.

Violence in Chicago grew to the point that 2016 was the bloodiest year the city had seen for two decades. Shootings spiked again during the summer of 2018; on one Sunday in August, forty-seven people were shot, including a stunning forty during a seven-hour period. Just a few days later, Mayor Emanuel decided not to seek reelection, a decision that rocked the city.

Cure Violence can be part of the solution to urban violence, but not on its own. The program addresses the symptoms of violence as well as some of its immediate causes, but the underlying factors that lead to violence remain. Those factors are in fact the same ones discussed earlier in this chapter—structural racism with deep historical roots, lack of economic opportunities, poor education, the lack of vibrant communities. Addressing violence, like any epidemic disease, in a comprehensive way demands both immediate and longer-term efforts. Otherwise the problem will keep coming back to plague the city, just as cholera did during much of its early development.

At Kaiser Permanente, we are applying the techniques in a different way. What can a large integrated health system do to prevent gun violence? Suicides account for nearly two-thirds of firearm deaths in the United States, and access to a gun increases the risk of suicide threefold. We must address firearm injuries as we do cancer, heart disease, and other leading causes of death in America.

Kaiser Permanente is funding studies to help us understand how to identify people at risk for intentional and unintentional firearm injuries, as well as exploring strategies to encourage at-risk people to store firearms more safely. This kind of predictive modeling is a key element in precision community health, as we explore in depth in chapter 4.

This is a promising line of research. Yet it is clear that precision community health does not have all the answers to these problems. I had hoped that our work in Chicago to reform mental health clinics and reduce violence would be more successful. Both efforts made me think hard about how I engaged with the diverse communities and institutions that are deeply invested in public health. What if I had invested more time to build better relationships with community leaders, the unions, or the police department? Would those relationships have helped me better understand their needs and where they overlap or diverge? The answer is undoubtedly yes.

It was inevitable that we would have setbacks. But the lessons we learned were clear: targeting the right communities with the right interventions at the right time requires a sophisticated approach to data and data management. Yet while those skills are necessary, they are not sufficient. That is because of the second word in the phrase *precision community health*. Communities are complex enough to thwart even our most sophisticated algorithms. If we want to be more precise, we need to understand how to work with diverse communities and build coalitions that work.

CHAPTER 3

Building Coalitions

PLACE CLEARLY MATTERS FOR HEALTH. Where you live, we now know more clearly than ever before, plays a significant, some might say even outsize, role in determining how healthy you are. But place is not just a spot on a map, some address you can navigate to using turn-by-turn directions from your smartphone. Place is also not simply a question of material things, be it schools or churches or hospitals or public parks. Place, from the perspective of health, is not just a question of *where* but also of *who*. Who are your friends, neighbors, coworkers, clergy, doctors, nurses? How we interact with one another and how strong are the ties that bind us contribute to our sense of security and well-being and are also affected by where we live.[1] For precision community health to be more than just an interesting idea, it needs to see community as a fundamental component of place.

Where we live and who we live with do not just describe us as people; they are keys to understanding which communities will thrive in terms of health and which will struggle. Epidemiologists, sociologists, and public health professionals have increasingly sophisticated tools to tease apart the many factors that contribute to our overall well-being, and while definitive answers remain elusive, it is clear that we must account for the contribution that social context makes to health status.[2]

Today, with nearly 2.7 million residents, Chicago is the third most populous and among the most culturally diverse cities in the United States. That diversity brings enormous resilience, but it can make governing a challenge. Few things—the Michael Jordan–era Chicago Bulls, for one—bring the entire city together. But if no one thing connects all Chicagoans, there are countless social ties, some stronger than others, that make up the fabric of the city. Building on and reinforcing those ties will be key to improving public health, not only in Chicago but anywhere.

Chicago's public health challenges are repeated in countless places. The number of non-elderly Chicagoans without health-care coverage when I was commissioner of public health topped five hundred thousand, though with the advent of the Affordable Care Act, that number has fallen. But Chicago has seen a tremendous increase over the past decade in the prevalence of overweight and obese adolescents and adults: according to data from 2010 and 2011 from the Centers for Disease Control and Prevention (CDC), over 60 percent of adults in Chicago were overweight or obese, while children in Chicago were significantly more likely to be obese than other children in the United States.[3]

During my tenure at the Chicago Department of Public Health (CDPH), smoking and teen pregnancy were troubling issues for many residents of Chicago. Violence is another challenge for the city. Prevention is an issue Chicago must also address, especially for its students. Over the past five years, Chicago saw a 44 percent increase in the percentage of high school students who reported that they missed school because they felt unsafe at school or en route to it.

Healthy Chicago was intended to address all of those problems. It was, and remains, an ambitious agenda. Mayor Rahm Emanuel and I recognized early on that we could not achieve what we knew was needed without broad, even unprecedented, cooperation across many diverse communities. With all our modern communication technologies and advances in medical science, our success would begin with good, old-fashioned shoe leather: I had to hit the streets to see where coalitions already existed and where they were missing, and I had to work on making sure the necessary coalitions were being built. The good news is that coalition building is part of Chicago's DNA.

I did so with a growing awareness of some troubling statistics. For all its wealth, the United States is not the healthiest country on Earth. Even though they spend less than we do on health care, other highly developed countries in Europe and Asia do far better than the United States in measures of health at nearly every stage of life, and the gap is growing. Part of the problem, and the one that gets the most attention, particularly at election time, is insurance: the lack of adequate coverage and access to high-quality medical care for all of our residents, particularly for low-income populations.

We clearly need to do better. But as challenging, politically and economically, as health insurance reform is, that may be the easier part of the problem. More subtle, entrenched, and stubborn social and economic forces, mediated by behavior and geography, are actually far more important drivers of population health dynamics. Along with economic disparities are racial and ethnic disparities in health that remain persistently high in the United States, and premature mortality rates have increased during the past fifteen years for white adults at midlife.[4] None of those trends are acceptable or sustainable.

Healthy Chicago was the most aggressive assault on health disparities the city ever attempted. The initiative brought together stakeholders from around the metropolitan area to create a public health agenda and set priorities, such as curbing tobacco use and reducing obesity rates. It's important to point out that the stakeholders weren't just the usual suspects from the health-care community but also included nontraditional partners such as technology firms, philanthropic groups, and faith-based organizations. Healthy Chicago generated dozens of strategies to address its priorities, and it made its goals public as a way of inviting accountability.

This chapter describes how I learned my first lesson about big-city public health: little of lasting value gets done without strong relationships. Good intentions and smart plans only get the ball rolling. If you are to make a real difference in people's lives, those intentions and plans need to be repeatedly tested by the actual communities they are intended to serve.

Why Community?

Community is a word, like *home* and *health*, redolent with positive connotations. Almost everyone would agree that community is, at least in some sense, a good thing, but few could define it with any great confidence. As social creatures, we are instinctively attracted to the idea. But what exactly is a community?

It turns out to be surprisingly hard to pin down. The National Academies of Sciences, Engineering, and Medicine took up this question in 2017 when it formed the Committee on Community-Based Solutions to Promote Health Equity in the United States. I was a member of that committee, and I remember vividly the debates we had over how to define what a community is and how it shapes the health of those living within it. We settled on this: "Community is any configuration of individuals, families, and groups whose values, characteristics, interests, geography, or social relations unite them in some way."[5] But we took pains to point out that the word *community* denotes both the people living in a place and the place itself. So we focused on shared geography, that is, place, as a key component of community—in other words, community is defined as the people living in a place, such as a neighborhood. Therefore, a community-based solution to promote health equity is an action, policy, program, or law that is driven by the community (members), affects local factors that can influence health, and has the potential to advance progress.

Again and again we returned to the metaphor of the fishbowl to describe the relationship between an individual and the conditions in which the individual lives. As first proposed by Katherine Keyes and Sandro Galea in their textbook *Population Health Science*,[6] the metaphor is as simple as can be: if the bowl in which a fish lives is dirty, or the glass is cracked and the water is leaking, the fish will never reach its full health potential, no matter how determined the fish might be. The life of a person is clearly more complex than that of a fish, and a community is no lifeless container, yet the metaphor captures the basic message of community health: we can try to change individual behaviors with every ounce of our collective strength and we will still fall short without considering their broader context—the policies, forces, and actions that influence people's choices over a lifetime and, indeed, over generations.

The phrase that has become increasingly in vogue, particularly in academic circles, to describe these factors is *social determinants of health*: local, national, even global problems such as poverty, unemployment, poor education, inadequate housing, poor public transportation, exposure to violence, pollution, and climate change all play a part in shaping people's health. But not everyone is exposed to these factors in equal measure, and some are fortunate enough to avoid many of them altogether, often because they or their parents had the financial wherewithal and flexibility to live where they liked. From that rather obvious yet pernicious dynamic stems the whole range of inequities that plague public health across the United States and beyond.

The word *determinant* suggests that these factors are fixed and the outcomes inevitable. My experience, however, and that of many others, shows this is not the case. While the forces that shape our health have deep roots and long histories, and often stem from entrenched economic and political dynamics, they are not in fact intractable. Almost every community I have seen has now, or has the potential to develop, the collective strength necessary to shift these long-standing dynamics.

The work of the National Academies committee confirmed what I had seen in Chicago. Community assets can be built, leveraged, and modified to create a context to achieve health equity. Communities throughout the United States have prioritized addressing the root causes of poor health and are demonstrating how specific upstream strategies lead to better conditions.

Community health is still a relatively new idea. The CDC created an organizational unit for community health in 2011 to implement congressionally mandated programs, and the term itself began to appear in the context of state-based programs in the late 1970s and early 1980s,[7] but there was no great sense of urgency and little consensus about what a community health program would do. Still, a few principles were beginning to emerge. The first is right there in the name: to improve the health of communities we need to engage them in deep and meaningful ways in order to understand their needs and their priorities. Then we can bring to bear the best of public health science to craft the strategies appropriate to meeting those needs. Community health is fundamentally concerned with making it easier for people to make healthy choices where they live, learn, work, and play. That requires moving health care beyond the doctor's office or clinic, focusing in particular on reaching people who are most at risk and redressing problems of health and socioeconomic inequities.

Community health is also collaborative to its core, across both social sectors and academic disciplines. That means engaging neighbors, businesses, government agencies, academic researchers, and other stakeholders in developing a shared agenda for health. And the collaborations don't always need to be primarily about health care, or even about health care at all. Not every community faces clear-cut threats, such as a neighborhood downwind of a power plant with high rates of asthma or bronchitis, for example. Sometimes they just want safe places for their children to play, or more affordable housing, or better jobs.

One basic tool for community health is the community health assessment. It is not a new invention; almost anyone with training in public health, nursing, or social work at some point in their education had to conduct a community health assessment to learn about the needs and assets of a particular community. If you are going to serve a community, it obviously makes sense to have a formal process for documenting the strengths and weaknesses in that community. Chicago and other big-city health departments have routinely conducted community health assessments for years.

Such has not been the case everywhere. Until recently, there was no uniform national standard for public health departments to meet, no way to determine which were rigorous and which were lax. Doctors, nurses, pharmacists, and therapists of all kinds need to show they have all the necessary training and are licensed by state or federal bodies. This was not so for public health departments, which is ironic, given the sweep and impact of their responsibilities. That gap was not filled until 2007, with the creation of a nonprofit organization called the Public Health Accreditation Board. For the first time, public health departments could apply for formal recognition that they were committed to high performance and continuous improvement.

Community health assessments were central to the accreditation process. When we released Healthy Chicago in 2011, one of the strategies we identified was to obtain accreditation. It was part of our planning and how we actively monitored the health of our residents. We saw the need to monitor risk factors, and as a result we came up with an approach that allowed us to look at multiple issues at the same time.

Accreditation also helped push Chicago, and indeed the field of public health in general, in the direction of a precision approach. The first item in the Public Health Accreditation Board guidelines focuses almost exclusively on data: the collection, analysis, and dissemination of data; use of data to inform public health policies, processes, and interventions; and participation in a collaborative process for the development of a shared, comprehensive health assessment of the community.[8] The emphasis on the importance of data in public health could not be clearer.

We wanted to be the first big city to earn the credential. Jaime Dircksen at the CDPH led a team and worked tirelessly to get us there. It took us eighteen months, and in August 2013 we were excited to become the first big-city health department to be accredited in the United States.

Two key factors make accreditation successful: first, leadership and teamwork; and second, the lens through which we view the accreditation process. Leadership and teamwork must come from the top as well as from the staff's commitment. That creates an environment where the process will be a solid one. How we view accreditation is also important. Rather than an added burden, it becomes part of the health department's existing work—a way to build improvement into day-to-day activities and to document that progress.

Social Capital and Public Health

Assessments are an important tool for any public health department. But they are just one step toward understanding a community's social context and ultimately making it healthier. The compelling yet conceptually slippery notion of social capital is often used to evaluate how well a community functions. So it is worth examining when developing strategies to improve public health.

Social capital broadly refers to the relationships and shared norms—among them values, trust, cooperation, and reciprocity—that enable social groups to function. The most obvious manifestation of social capital is the ease with which people form themselves into groups of one sort or another. It was one of the defining characteristics of our country from its early days; in the 1830s, Alexis de Tocqueville used the phrase *the art of association* to describe Americans' propensity for civil association, which he saw as the cornerstone of the uniquely American form of democracy: "Americans of all ages, all stations in life, and all types of disposition are forever forming associations."

Tocqueville believed that associations were a feature of democracy. Without them, in an egalitarian society, people would be unable to bring about change or participate meaningfully in public life, hampered by a surfeit of individualism. Voluntary associations, both trivial and important, were the antidote, bringing communal strength to weak individuals. In Tocqueville's native France, in contrast, on the eve of the Revolution "there were not ten Frenchmen who could come together for a common cause." Neither Tocqueville nor anyone else at the time was much concerned with questions of public health, but the link between equality and social cohesion has reemerged as a vital concern for how to address modern problems of health and well-being.

The idea of social capital entered the field of sociology in the late 1980s, but it came to broad public attention through the work of Harvard University political scientist Robert Putnam, particularly his 2000 book *Bowling Alone*,[9] in which he described what he saw as the fraying of interpersonal bonds in American society and the parlous effects that would have on democracy.

Putnam saw a culture in which social capital was declining. If true, that trend would have ominous consequences, and not just for politics. The idea that more cohesive communities were also healthier was not new. The most famous example came from the eastern Pennsylvania town of Roseto, which in the 1950s was a close-knit, largely immigrant community of about sixteen hundred people. Roseto caught the attention of two medical researchers, Stewart Wolf and John G. Bruhn, because of a curious fact: residents of Roseto were to all appearances much like the people in neighboring towns—they smoked as much, were just as overweight, were just as likely to be sedentary, and ate the same diet—yet they were much less likely to have a heart attack.

The biggest difference between Roseto and its neighbors had nothing to do with the typical risk factors that physicians look for. It had to do with culture and the behaviors and attitudes that come with it. The first people to settle in Roseto in the 1880s had come largely from the village of Roseto Valfortore in Apulia, the rural, relatively poor region that makes up the heel of Italy's boot. They brought with them both tight bonds and a deep-seated—and socially enforced—egalitarianism and aversion to ostentation and conspicuous consumption.

Then, in the 1960s, Roseto began to change, and as it did, the town became the setting for a natural experiment in public health that could never be carried out in any other way. Once insular, Roseto inevitably began to yield to the sweep of American culture. Young people began to move away to seek jobs in neighboring towns, and as they did, Roseto's social bonds began to weaken. Wolf and Bruhn continued to track the health of the town's residents, and they found that within a decade, the incidence of heart attack in Roseto had caught up with that of neighboring towns.[10]

Roseto was far from the only example of the phenomenon. In 1897, sociologist Émile Durkheim found that social integration, or the lack of it, was a key element in differing suicide rates in various communities.[11] In 1965, Lester Breslow was one of the principal investigators in a landmark long-term study in Alameda County, California, that assessed the effects of daily habits and social relationships on physical and mental health. They identified a suite of behaviors key to good health that would become known as the Alameda 7 and are now nearly universal: eat regular meals, including breakfast; get seven to eight hours of sleep; maintain a healthy weight; do not smoke; limit your alcohol consumption; and get regular physical activity. That all seems obvious now, but it was far from obvious at the time.[12]

Even less obvious was what emerged from a nine-year study of the same cohort.[13] That study found that those with few social ties were two to three times more likely to die of all causes than were those with more extensive contacts. That observation was important for physicians concerned with treating individual patients, but less so from the perspective of public health. The connection between social capital and well-being across entire communities had not yet been made because the mechanism by which social capital would impact public health, for good or ill, had not been explored. But its time was coming.

The idea of social capital is powerful, but it is not perfect. For one thing, it is difficult, if not impossible, to measure with any real confidence. Robert Putnam took a fairly straightforward approach by counting groups in civil society—sports clubs, bowling leagues, literary societies, political clubs, and the like—and tracking their memberships over time and across different geographic regions. There are other, more mathematically sophisticated measures, but there is still no consensus on the best method, in no small part because there is no practical way to attach a number to something such as trust or cohesion and expect that a majority of people would agree that it is the right number.

If social capital is like other kinds of capital, there is also the question of how we might create more of it and whether more social capital is always what we want. After all, as political scientist Francis Fukuyama pointed out, the Ku Klux Klan has an abundance of social capital and cohesion.[14] But the general sense is that more cohesion and more trust are good things, and that is certainly the case in terms of public health.

So how, exactly, is social capital tied to public health? There are a number of plausible mechanisms. One line of research brings the impact all the way down to the biophysical level, demonstrating measurable impacts on our immune systems, neural networks, respiratory systems, and so on. That work dates back at least two decades, and there is now a rich body of research that supports the idea that our social context has real physical manifestations.[15]

That is a fascinating and important finding on many levels, but it does not get at the importance of social capital for the health of entire communities. For that, we need to look more broadly at how varying levels of social capital translate into behaviors that influence health status. Are people in areas with low social capital, for example, less likely to exercise, or more likely to commit or be victims of violent crime? Research into both of those questions suggests the answer is yes.[16]

One troubling hypothesis from a public health perspective is that a lack of social capital may make it harder for certain groups to get access to health care. One study of twenty-two metropolitan statistical areas in the United States found that residents in communities with higher levels of social capital reported fewer problems in accessing health care.[17] Another found that communities high in social capital were able to provide better service integration and housing, though not better clinical outcomes, to homeless people with severe mental illness.[18]

Income inequality, as we have seen, is a key element in health inequity as well. One of the ways income inequality damages health is by weakening social bonds in poor communities. Another study, published in 1997, looked across thirty-nine states and measured civic engagement by per capita membership in groups or associations, and trust in others based on responses to two questions specifically inquiring about fairness and trust. Low levels of group membership and high levels of mistrust were found to correlate with higher mortality rates. The primary effect of income inequality on mortality was mediated by the level of social capital; lack of wealth alone was not strongly correlated with higher rates of mortality. While there are many studies linking social integration to health in individuals, this study was the first to demonstrate a link between mortality and social capital at the population level. The important interpretation was that low social capital is one way that income inequality threatens the health of an entire community.[19]

Building Social and Public Health Capital in Chicago

Social capital clearly plays a role in public health, but it may be indirect, and as a practitioner, it was unclear to me when I became commissioner in Chicago how I might help build the social capital of the city's diverse neighborhoods. But there is a related concept that is more tangible, at least if you are looking at the problem from the trenches. If we can build robust, collaborative partnerships across business, government, social service organizations, community groups, and so on, we can build what Glen Mays and his colleagues at the University of Kentucky call "comprehensive population health system capital."[20]

That's an unlovely phrase, but the reasoning beneath it is compelling. It is increasingly evident that addressing a wide range of behavioral, social, economic, and environmental challenges requires an equally broad set of public health activities: assessing population health status and needs, educating the public about health risks and prevention strategies, engaging community stakeholders in planning and implementing health improvement strategies, and linking individuals to health and social services, while at the same time protecting the quality and safety of water, food, air, housing, and the physical environment.

There is also compelling evidence of the benefits of public health programs that target such risk factors as smoking, diet, physical activity, and substance abuse and that address unmet needs for housing, education, and so on. Recent analyses suggest that lowering these risk factors to optimal levels among US residents could reduce the racial and geographic disparities observed in cardiovascular disease and diabetes mortality by 69–80 percent and the disparities observed in cancer mortality by 29–50 percent.[21]

No single government agency, in fact no government writ large, can tackle those challenges alone. This is not news; public health in the United States has always been a collaborative effort of state and local public health agencies and community organizations supported by a mix of public and private resources. What has changed is our understanding of the scale of the challenge and hence the scale of the collaboration that is needed.

Our public health infrastructure, like physical infrastructure of roads, bridges, sewers, and schools, is in dire need of repair and renovation. And as with physical infrastructure, the money for those repairs can be hard to find amid a patchwork of federal, state, local, and private funding streams with distinct target populations, eligibility criteria, service providers, and implementation requirements.

One approach to solving the problem, and one Mayor Emanuel and I built into the foundation of the Healthy Chicago plan, was to form multi-sector partnerships to coordinate the delivery of health and social services. We were building on a rich history of innovations aimed at reducing risk factors, decreasing disease and injury, and promoting health.[22]

The importance of partnerships had been clear to me since I began working at Heartland Alliance for Human Needs & Human Rights. At that time, I was a practicing family physician at the Health Care for the Homeless program in Chicago. I remember one night when I was talking to people at a homeless shelter and I met a man who was spending his first night on the street. I began talking to him about screening for hypertension, diabetes, and colorectal cancer. He looked at me and asked, "What don't you get? I'm worried about where I am going to sleep tomorrow, or get my next meal." Cancer screening, important as it is, was not on his radar, and for good reason.

That brought home the reality of community health. Who will house the homeless, feed the hungry, find jobs for the jobless? All of that obviously matters profoundly for the health of individuals and the communities of which they are a part, but is beyond the scope of any single public health institution. It is the partnerships we form that will help give this person the chance to thrive.

The challenge became even clearer at the CDPH, when I began to think about the nearly 3 million people in the city. We faced the same set of problems at a bigger scale. I am also seeing similar challenges at Kaiser Permanente. Every day, 12.4 million people across the United States trust us with their care and coverage needs. We estimate that about 3.5 million members are living below 250 percent of the federal poverty level (FPL) (that is just over $12,000 for individuals and $25,000 for a family of four). That puts those people at significant risk of hunger, homelessness, inadequate transportation, and social isolation—the same issues I saw when speaking to the homeless man in a shelter fifteen years ago. Even more troubling, over 1.5 million of the Kaiser Permanente members living below 250 percent of the FPL are commercially insured, which means they get insurance through their employers, so even with jobs, they still face significant social health risks.

The public health community loves the idea of partnerships because they work. The risk, and something I saw over and over again in town hall meetings and other forums, is that just creating partnerships and making plans is the easy part; the more challenging and more important part is making those plans actionable. State agencies, institutes, and think tanks can take five years to develop a five-year plan, and then it is time to start the next cycle. That obviously gets us nowhere.

The point was driven home in early 2019 when I participated in a congressional hearing on housing and health. Congressman Jim McGovern of Massachusetts said that while plans were all well and good, what he needed was something he could act on now. Even the most compelling plan is worthless if it just sits on shelves gathering dust.

That was a key reason why we were determined to develop Healthy Chicago as quickly as we could, which meant understanding that the first iteration of the plan would not be perfect. We made sure that the plan included the mechanisms needed to show where we were on achieving our goals, so we could adjust as needed.

In the early 1970s, researchers in California and Finland independently took that approach when they decided to test the hypothesis that community-wide programs to change individual behavior could lead to improvements in cardiovascular health. The fascinating thing in both cases is that the studies were designed as experiments, with interventions and controls.[23] That was groundbreaking, and when the results showed that public health campaigns could indeed change behavior, the interest in community health exploded. More studies followed, including a five-city study in California that began in 1978 and continued for six years, exposing thousands of people to public service announcements, television programs, newspaper columns, and other materials designed to inspire heart-healthy behaviors and diets. As with the earlier studies, the Stanford Five-City Project demonstrated that a community-based approach held great promise for solving some long-standing public health problems.[24]

In the United States, the federal government soon began exploring the idea. The CDC launched the Planned Approach to Community Health (PATCH) program in the early 1980s, and it was just the first of many national efforts.[25] Local, nongovernmental, community-based organizations and programs also began springing up around the country.

The momentum for community health was clearly growing, but it was not until the passage of the Affordable Care Act (ACA), which became law a little more than a year before we announced Healthy Chicago, that things really took off. The ACA established new incentives for hospitals, health insurers, public health agencies, and employers to contribute to community-wide health programs, nudging these sectors toward greater coordination and collaboration.

In 2010, the CDC, for example, created the Communities Putting Prevention to Work (CPPW) program to reduce illness, death, and the economic burden of chronic diseases. Over three years, the CDC spent more than $400 million across fifty communities—including Chicago—and 55 million people to prevent obesity and reduce tobacco use and exposure to secondhand smoke. Nationwide, according to one study, the investment in community health and prevention policy may prevent thousands of premature deaths and save the nation billions of dollars. The study found that the CPPW investment in prevention efforts could avert fourteen thousand premature deaths, $2.4 billion in discounted direct medical costs, and $9.5 billion in discounted lifetime and annual productivity losses between 2010 and 2020.[26]

I knew how transformative those grants would be. The CPPW was in the works at the same time as Healthy Chicago, and both were being built on the understanding that community health efforts would be fundamental to long-term changes in behavior that would benefit the health of all residents. I also knew that the challenge before us in Chicago was to connect the growing interest in community health with my desire, and the mayor's, to bring a new precision to our approach.

Building coalitions across a diverse city, especially coalitions designed to change things as personal as diet and lifestyle, might be seen as the opposite of precise. Coalitions are almost by definition messy, sometimes contentious, and almost always full of both passion and negotiation.

Healthy Chicago was tied directly to the precision approach. Our goal was to identify those who are most disenfranchised and provide them with the support to lift themselves up. The flip side of that is as obvious as it is controversial: Healthy Chicago was not, in the first instance, about lifting all boats simultaneously. That is just not possible.

We knew when we launched the first version of the plan that we had to target the most vulnerable communities. That was the easy part. Then we had to get out and listen to what those communities had to say. It was not always easy to hear. Some people were upset that their priorities were not included in Healthy Chicago. As important as autism is, for example, it never made it to the top twelve priorities for the city. I heard from many mothers that this was an oversight. We simply couldn't include all issues. We had to be realistic about what we could achieve.

Partnership development and collaboration are key to making Healthy Chicago work. I set a challenge in Chicago that if your organization's logo is not on the slide I share when we talk about partnerships, then we need to talk. Improving the health of Chicago is about pushing the envelope and making those partnerships as strong as they can be by respecting, listening to, and learning from all the coalition members. At the same time, it was the role of the CDPH to support all the partners with the best possible data so that progress would be based on evidence. We wanted to foster equity, to lift up the voices of the community, while also bringing important information to the table. The tricky part is finding the right balance of providing information without instructing the communities on what they should consider important.

There are many examples of critical partners who are helping to improve public health in Chicago. We worked with fifteen city agencies to make Healthy Chicago a success story. For example, working with the Chicago Department of Transportation, we brought more than thirty-five miles of protected bike lanes to the city, along with more than three thousand bikes and three hundred bike share stations throughout the city, providing an added mode of transportation and physical activity.

With the help of Blue Cross Blue Shield of Illinois and Local Initiatives Support Corporation (LISC) Chicago—the local office of the nation's leading community development support organization—we developed the PlayStreets program. On a regular basis, Chicago blocks off streets in the city so parents and kids can get out and be active, with activities such as taking a Zumba class and playing with Hula-Hoops.

We partnered with the GE Foundation, Northwestern University, and Mile Square Health Center in Chicago, identified two neighborhoods with the highest rates of cardiovascular disease, and started doing mass screenings. Such partnerships were critical to advance Healthy Chicago.

Other extraordinary partnerships already existed, and we were able to build on their work to achieve dramatic results. The Metropolitan Chicago Breast Cancer Task Force, for example, was created in 2007 in response to disturbing reports that black women in Chicago were far more likely than white women to die from breast cancer. The Task Force's own study confirmed the data: black women were in fact 68 percent more likely than white women to die from breast cancer, compared with 11 percent in New York City and 37 percent nationwide.[27] After meeting with the Task Force, it was clear that we had a path to really making a difference regarding breast cancer: we had the coalition, we had the data, and we had evidence of what worked in terms of prevention, screening, diagnosis, and treatment.

Working with the Task Force, the CDPH helped implement a series of steps to improve access to care, improve the quality of mammograms across the city—black women were much less likely to have their tests read by a breast cancer specialist—provide education about breast cancer and breast cancer screening, and help patients navigate the health system. As a result, between 1999 and 2013, the mortality rate from breast cancer among African American women in Chicago decreased by 13.9 percent. The disparity between African American and white women was reduced by more than 20 percent during the same time frame.[28]

That is a tremendous success story, but it also highlights the ongoing challenges of addressing health equity. The latest version of the mayor's plan, Healthy Chicago 2.0, was released in March 2016 and explicitly places equity at the heart of the matter. Indeed, the tagline for the plan is as clear as can be: Partnering to Improve Health Equity.

Building coalitions is not just a local task. We realized as we were laying out plans to address obesity, teen pregnancy, smoking, and other challenges that we would need a broader set of coalitions as well. We would have to think nationally. So we worked with other big cities to reinvigorate the Big Cities Health Coalition to collaborate with our peers across the country.

We also discovered that we needed new kinds of coalitions. We would have to work with faith-based communities, the philanthropy community, the information technology community, the business sector. Few of these typically have public health concerns at the top of their agenda, and some, particularly some big corporations, are actively at odds with what we are trying to accomplish. Deciding whom to work with and how is a big part of precision community health.

The most important lesson I learned from this work is that partnerships are absolutely fundamental to improving the health of a community. In Chicago it didn't happen overnight, but we eventually had enough partners standing with us to help achieve our goals. It's all about developing a culture that has public health as top priority. For the tobacco prevention campaign (which is discussed in detail in chapter 5), for example, we worked with the American Lung Association and Respiratory Health Association. For obesity, we worked closely with CLOCC—the Consortium to Lower Obesity in Chicago Children. We worked closely with Blue Cross Blue Shield and with the Chicago Park District and the Active Transportation Alliance. We built a long list of engaged partners to make a difference.

The use of coalitions can achieve things that other tactics cannot. Shortly after Mayor Emanuel took office, for example, he set a goal of cutting by half the city's food deserts—neighborhoods without healthy food outlets—by the end of his first term. He gathered chief executives from major grocery chains and pushed them to put stores in underserved communities. That was important, but it was not enough. I knew we needed a coalition-based approach to the problem of obesity in the city.

A few years earlier, Dr. Katherine Christoffel, a pediatrician with Northwestern University's Feinberg School of Medicine, had brought together a group of organizations interested in addressing this issue and started CLOCC. Kathy had the insight and the courage to bring people together, and she started a movement in Chicago. I got to work with Kathy over the years, and I learned a lot from her. Together with CLOCC, we engaged community organizers to work with ten shopkeepers in Englewood, South Chicago, and Humboldt Park to bring healthy food into their stores. Corner stores can be part of the food-desert problem when all they stock is candy and chips. They can be part of the solution when they sell fresh fruit and vegetables.

If we could make healthy food an easy and affordable option, we could take a big step toward addressing the obesity epidemic. We had learned from our violence prevention work that we needed to address not just the symptom—overweight children and adults—but also the underlying causes. That meant reversing a cultural shift that began more than fifty years ago, when diets began changing from fresh, nutrient-rich foods to processed foods, sugary drinks, and fried snacks.

Working closely with CLOCC, we developed a plan to improve the nutrition of residents and workers by targeting the physical and cultural environments in which food is sold, marketed, and consumed. We found that the most effective way to address obesity and related diseases is to change the day-to-day environment so that it supports healthy eating while discouraging the consumption of unhealthy foods.[29]

We had also learned from the mental health reform effort that we needed to be far more inclusive. The plan was unique because of its obesity prevention focus, hybrid public health and community planning framework, and inclusive design process, with both government and nongovernmental participation. The recommendations were the result of a comprehensive public planning process that included more than two dozen public meetings involving more than four hundred individuals held over thirteen months to gather feedback.

More and more people, at every level of public health, were making meaningful investments in a multisector community health approach. We had good reason to believe it should work, and anecdotal evidence was accumulating that it did work. It wasn't until after I left Chicago that we began to see conclusive data that supported that intuition.

In 2016, Glen Mays and his colleagues[30] examined sixteen years' worth of data from the Robert Wood Johnson Foundation's National Longitudinal Survey of Public Health Systems, which follows a national cohort of US communities over time, measuring the scope of health programs in each community and the range of organizations involved. Using this and other sources of data, they evaluated whether these activities reduced community mortality rates.

The findings show the value of creating dense multisector networks. The largest health improvements associated with system capital were observed for deaths from causes that are largely preventable, including cardiovascular disease, diabetes, and influenza. This is one of the best pieces of evidence that engaging diverse groups in health planning translates into tangible results.

An interesting question is how exactly the partnerships we built in Chicago lead to the kinds of health improvements that Mays and his colleagues documented. We might not be able to demonstrate a direct cause-and-effect relationship. What we saw, and the Mays study confirmed, was that communities with comprehensive systems were significantly more likely than their counterparts to adopt comprehensive smoking bans, and they achieved lower rates of smoking, obesity, and physical inactivity among low-income residents. Higher levels of system capital may help communities change policy and social and environmental conditions—such as access to recreation opportunities, healthy food, and community exercise groups—that improve health for at-risk populations.

The trends are positive, but we are still falling far short. As of 2014, almost 40 percent of US metropolitan communities had built the kind of the networks that are associated with reduced mortality.[31] That's good news, since in 1998 the figure was a mere 24 percent. On the other hand, the data are a sobering reminder of how far we have to go: less than half of the country provides its residents with what we really should consider a basic level of health infrastructure, both physical and social.

That infrastructure rests on the strength of local partnerships. Without them it would be nearly impossible to understand the priorities of the communities we need to reach. While coalition building seems unrelated to our digital world, it is in fact fundamental to precision community health. Partnerships allow us to take advantage of the power of big data in ways that we would never have imagined just a few years ago.

CHAPTER 4

Tapping the Power of Big Data

Do you remember the Zika virus? It would not be all that surprising if the answer were no. Public memory is short; unless you are among those unfortunate enough to have been directly affected by this devastating illness, the details may have faded as quickly as the headlines. But in 2015 and 2016, the fear was palpable. Travel advisories went up, and many pregnant women decided not to go to Rio de Janeiro for the 2016 Summer Olympics. Congress became embroiled in a fierce debate over how much money to spend on combating the Zika virus.

Lost in the blur of numbers was a more pressing question: Can we predict where the next outbreak will be? Anticipating, rather than simply responding to, crises such as Zika, or the lead poisoning in Flint, Michigan, is the next leap in improving public health here and around the world.

Fortunately, new technologies are making it easier to address health problems before they become epidemics. Big data, predictive analytics, and social networking all offer invaluable opportunities for innovation. If we are willing to use them, these tools can improve the health of the growing number of people living in the new megacities that dot every continent and will increasingly shape the global environment.

Scientists have been aware of the potential power of being able to analyze trillions of bytes of data from many sources since the 1990s or even earlier, long before computers could even store that much information. Few outside the tech community, however, knew much about the idea until about 2010, as our ability to store, communicate, and analyze data exploded.[1] The term *big data* does not refer only to a large quantity of data; it is an idea that also includes diverse sources of data and data that are being generated at a heretofore unimaginable frequency and speed. We are, all of us, now creating data constantly—where we go and how many steps we take to get there, what we buy and how often, how many calories we consume and how many we burn. It is a frightening prospect on the one hand, with profound implications for privacy, security, and even democracy. But the potential to generate new insights into how we live and to use those insights to improve our health are powerful as well.

With the advent of computers powerful enough to process such data sets, people began to see opportunities to leverage big data everywhere they looked. Not surprisingly, big corporations were among the first to jump on the bandwagon. Companies such as Amazon and Walmart began using big data to understand their customers better and therefore market their products more effectively.

The public health community is beginning to take a page from this commercial playbook, using big data to understand populations better. While data collection has always been part of public health practice, new technologies allow us to make associations and comparisons in ways that were not possible using standard analytics.

The potential of big data became clear to me in 2012 when I was meeting with a group of data scientists from Allstate, one of the largest insurance companies in the world. It occurred to me that if you apply for car insurance with just about any reputable company in the country, you will face a battery of questions: your age, occupation, and marital status; the kind of car you drive, how far you drive, and for what purpose; your driving record; and so on.

I asked the data scientists why they collected such detailed data. "It's obvious," they said. "We have built algorithms that assess all the factors that go into determining the risk that a driver will be in a car accident, and we use that assessment to set that driver's insurance rate."

At that moment I realized something else that was just as obvious but that I had never noticed. I asked if they could use the same approach to come up with an algorithm to help us determine which restaurants in the city were at risk of health code violations.

"Of course we can," they said. Then they said something that really hit home. "You mean you don't do that already?"

Surveillance in the Age of Data

It was embarrassing but true. The way Chicago and most other major cities track health code violations, the presence of lead in homes or water supplies, and other threats to public health was woefully outdated. Public health departments have always collected information, or "conducted surveillance," on their populations. But they have often been resistant to innovation, and approaches to surveillance have not always kept up with the times.

Over their long history, public health departments have used all manner of methods to collect these data. The early focus was on epidemic diseases, and surveillance amounted to a person-by-person record of who was sick and with whom they had been in contact. The issues on which data were needed gradually expanded, and in 1872 the newly founded American Public Health Association (APHA), as one of its first acts, sent out a survey to every town of more than five thousand inhabitants with questions on virtually everything of concern to public health, including the towns' elevation, miles of paved streets, ventilation of public buildings, cleanliness of the water supply, and adequacy (or existence) of sewer systems.[2]

The survey was a first, but it was not a smashing success. Many of those who received it were unable or unwilling to respond. While the founding of the APHA was a landmark event in the development of public health as a profession, the fact remained that public health officials' ability to collect and make use of vital statistics was haphazard at best.

The sophistication of data collection methods, as well as the commitment on the part of governments to invest the resources needed to make the collection consistent and reliable, continued to grow throughout the twentieth century. But the explosion of computing power in the past ten years or so has changed the game entirely. Seemingly overnight, anyone had access to computers with the processing speed and memory to handle massive amounts of data.

One of the first applications of computer technology to health care emerged from an innovative program at Kaiser Permanente in the 1950s. At the time, health plans did not provide health checkups unless one had a medical complaint. But Lester Breslow, then at the California Department of Public Health in Berkeley, argued for the screening of healthy populations, particularly industrial workers. Kaiser Permanente had originally covered only the employees of Henry J. Kaiser's shipyards during World War II, but by the 1950s it was also expanding to serve the public, particularly unions such as the International Longshore and Warehouse Union (ILWU).

Working with Breslow, the US Public Health Service, the California Department of Health and other public health agencies, and physicians at Kaiser Permanente developed an integrated battery of preliminary examinations—what Breslow termed a "multiphasic screening examination."[3] The first group test was conducted at the ILWU's Local 10 hall at Pier 18 in San Francisco and screened several thousand longshoremen. It was a groundbreaking step for public health and preventive medicine.

The process consisted of about fifteen procedures—blood and urine tests, chest X-ray, electrocardiogram, and so on—but required the presence of only a single physician, assisted by paramedics, thus keeping costs low. By the mid-1950s, 30 to 40 percent of all new Kaiser Permanente members were choosing the multiphasic exam on their first visit.

The tests generated mountains of health records—including information on 170 occupational titles and a battery of work-related health questions—all of which were collected and maintained manually. That was, of course, standard practice, as there were no readily available alternatives, but the sheer amount of information was unprecedented. Never before had so many healthy people taken so many medical tests in such a short period of time.

By the early 1960s, computers were sufficiently advanced to enable the automation of health records for the first time. In 1961, the US Public Health Service awarded the Kaiser Foundation Research Institute a grant to study automation of the multiphasic health testing. Members would now go through the screening stations with computer punch cards that got marked along the way. At the end of the session, which took a couple of hours, there would now be a computerized medical record of their current health status.

The results were analyzed in bulk by computer, which allowed doctors to spot trends in community health and work to address public health risks. It was the beginning of a new era.

Dr. Morris F. Collen, one of the seven founding physicians of The Permanente Medical Group (TPMG), was the driving force behind the effort and one of the early pioneers of medical informatics. In 1966 he presciently noted that "the advent of automation and computers may introduce a new era of preventive medicine."[4] Dr. Collen would later predict that the computer would probably have the greatest technological impact on medical science since the invention of the microscope.[5]

Medical informatics has spawned innumerable efforts to harness computers to help with such tasks as automating medical charts, linking laboratory data to clinical data, computerized diagnostic systems, biomedical engineering, and so on. Many of these efforts were intended to improve the efficiency and hence reduce the cost of health care.

Public health informatics began to take shape in the 1990s, applying the new tools of the information age to the age-old problems of public health. By one early definition, public health informatics is "the application of information science and technology to public health practice and research."[6] In practice, bringing the two fields—so different in history, mission, and approach—together demands innovation on both sides. In addition to using the wealth of computing power at everyone's fingertips, we needed to shift the mind-set of public health professionals, for many of whom informatics was more than a new tool; it was an entirely new language. It was clear to me in Chicago that if we were to take full advantage of the information revolution, we would need more than new and better software, faster processors, and more elaborate pocket computers that we occasionally use to make a phone call. We needed fundamentally new ways of thinking about the practice of public health.

A major driver of the informatics revolution was the 2009 Health Information Technology for Economic and Clinical Health (HITECH) Act, which was intended to reimburse health-care providers for using electronic health records systems.[7] We worked with a key partner, the Chicago Health Information Technology Regional Extension Center, to make progress on electronic health records surveillance for population health. The HealthLNK Data Repository is a database of de-identified health records data for Chicagoans. It encompasses inpatient and outpatient visits spanning five years. Furthermore, individual patient records are matched across institutions. This work resulted in support from the Patient-Centered Outcomes Research Institute (PCORI) to twenty institutions across Chicago to build a clinical data research network to advance population health. This network is part of a larger PCORI network effort. This endeavor helped drive new insights in population health for Chicago.

The other obvious application of computing power to questions of medicine and public health is to sequencing and analyzing DNA. It makes sense. Our genome is an astonishing mine of information that captures everything from our deep evolutionary history to our possible future health: Do I have genes that put me at risk for heart disease or cancer? Big data technologies gave researchers new ways to sequence and analyze the billions of base pairs in the human genome in search of clues about infections, cancer, and noncommunicable diseases. Disease researchers now also have access to human genetic data and genomic databases of millions of bacteria—data they can combine to study treatment outcomes.

It is a powerful new tool, and the prospects for improving medical practice are dramatic indeed. In May 2018, the National Institutes of Health launched its All of Us campaign, which aims to conduct detailed genetic studies of one million US volunteers over a ten-year period at a cost of $1.45 billion. The project promises to "lay the scientific foundation for a new era of personalized, highly effective health care."

The idea that emerging technologies can tell us who is vulnerable to which disease is the basis of the precision public health approach advocated by Muin J. Khoury, head of the Office of Genomics and Precision Public Health at the Centers for Disease Control and Prevention (CDC), and others (see the introduction for more on the distinction between precision public health and precision community health).

There are caveats, of course. Too great a focus on the genetic aspects of health could, for example, undermine attention to the broader social determinants of health, particularly income and racial inequalities.[8]

We are already seeing the first application of genomics in a community setting. The MyCode Community Health Initiative is a precision medicine project of the Geisinger Health Plan, a provider serving parts of Pennsylvania and New Jersey. MyCode analyzes the DNA of patient-participants who sign up. More than two hundred thousand patient-participants were signed up by mid-2018. More than five hundred Geisinger MyCode participants have received clinical reports telling them that they have a genomic variant that increases their risk of early cancers or heart disease, allowing their doctors to detect and treat these conditions before any clinical symptoms become present.

But the potential public health uses of big data extend well beyond genomics. In 2016, the Bill & Melinda Gates Foundation hosted a conference titled "Precision Public Health: The First 1,000 Days," which focused on how data analysis and visualization may reinvigorate public health surveillance. The central idea was that big data of many different types could be employed to make health care more precise, benefiting everyone.[9] At some point, precision public health and precision community health will likely converge. Ten years from now, or even sooner than that, your genome may be central to serving you and your community. The more genomics and public health data technology evolve, the closer they'll come.

We also need to be able to compare, for example, the wealth of data on environmental factors such as pollution with the rich data on respiratory disease. There are vast, largely untapped streams of data about individuals' social networks and behaviors that could help us understand how diseases spread and how we might stop them, or at least find ways to alert us when an epidemic outbreak might be on the horizon.

All of this raises significant concerns about privacy. When personal health information was held in handwritten notes in the file cabinets of countless medical offices around the country, the risk of large-scale data theft was effectively zero. Digitization has utterly changed that situation. Data breaches, including those at major insurance companies, are becoming regular occurrences. One of the worst breaches occurred in

May 2019, when hackers broke into the data networks of blood-testing groups Quest Diagnostics, LabCorp, and Opko Health and stole the personal information of twenty million customers.

The most significant law governing medical data is the Health Insurance Portability and Accountability Act (HIPAA), which President Bill Clinton signed into law in 1996. The law required the secretary of the Department of Health and Human Services to create regulations to protect the privacy and security of health information—prior to HIPAA there was no general set of national security standards to protect health information.

HIPAA will likely need to be updated to account for developments in new health-care technologies and practices. Both government regulators and patients have good reason to be concerned that the proliferation of new sources of personal data means that the risk of exposure is growing as well. One critical question is whether lawmakers will see health data as just one aspect of the larger issue of data privacy in the internet age or whether medical data offer unique challenges that will lead to calls for stand-alone legislation.

There is also big money at stake with big data. According to McKinsey & Company, with the right tools, big data could be worth nine billion dollars to US public health surveillance alone by improving detection of and response to infectious disease outbreaks and three hundred billion dollars to American health care in general through reductions in expenditures.[10]

With so much money on the table, there is also the risk that health data will be misused even if the data are acquired legally. According to a report by ProPublica and National Public Radio, data brokers are gathering and selling personal details about hundreds of millions of Americans.[11] Although HIPAA covers medical data, the companies are casting a far wider net, tracking data on race, education level, television-viewing habits, marital status, net worth, social media activity, what you buy, and whether you pay your bills. Airlines are collecting more and more biometric data as part of expediting security screening processes. All of this information feeds into algorithms that identify you and that can spit out predictions about how much your health care could cost.

Using such lifestyle data to make inferences about possible future health-care needs poses both medical and ethical challenges. Medically, such data are rife with errors, and the links between any particular behavior and an illness are often tenuous at best. The good news is that the Affordable Care Act (ACA) prohibits insurers from denying people coverage on the basis of preexisting health conditions or charging sick people more for individual or small group plans. The future of the law, however, remains very much an open question.

Other countries are testing alternatives to addressing the problem. In May 2019, a strict law called the General Data Protection Regulation went into effect in Europe and made data protection a fundamental right.

Learning

In 1999, the Institute of Medicine (renamed the National Academy of Medicine in 2015) began to develop an idea called the Learning Health-care System. The first report from the initiative was titled *To Err Is Human*, and the key finding was disturbing: an estimated 44,000 to 98,000 Americans may die annually as a result of medical errors. That would rank medical errors as one of the top ten leading killers if such errors were considered a formal cause of death.[12] The fact is, until relatively recently, most physicians did not focus much effort on analyzing the scientific evidence on what is effective and under what circumstances. Sometimes the data do not exist; sometimes they exist but are hard to find; and sometimes doctors are not convinced that changing their approaches to treatment will actually lead to better outcomes for their patients.

The idea of evidence-based medicine emerged in the twentieth century as a response to these trends. The goal was to improve care by integrating individual clinical expertise with the best available external evidence.[13] It marked a significant advance, and it highlights the importance of both a rigorous scientific base for practice and physician judgment. However, the increased complexity of health care requires a deepened commitment to examining evidence relevant to the treatment of individual patients.

This is not to suggest that physicians have anything less than their patients' interests at heart. Far from it. The fact is that most simply can't keep up with the pace of new discoveries, new data, and new ways of thinking about how to make the best possible clinical decisions. We can hardly blame them for that. Ask most practicing physicians what they need most, and they'll tell you it is to spend more time with their patients. Yet they could spend literally every waking hour immersed in the details of new scientific knowledge, including about disease management, medical technologies, regenerative medicine, and the growing utility of genomics and proteomics in tailoring disease detection and treatment to each individual. The amount of research is vast, and currently the share of health expenses devoted to determining what works best is about one-tenth of 1 percent.[14]

By the early 2000s, it was becoming clear that an evidence-based approach was not sufficient by itself and certainly had little impact on public health. What was needed was a wholesale change in the development and application of evidence for health care. The Institute of Medicine led the effort, recognizing the role that information technology could play by improving data collection and management. But the Institute wanted to go beyond that to conduct a thorough reevaluation of how health care is structured to develop and apply evidence—from health professions training to infrastructure development, patient engagement, payments, and measurement. As the Institute said in its 2007 report, "The nation needs a healthcare system that learns."[15]

The Institute of Medicine's Learning Healthcare System was a platform that allowed evidence-based real-time analysis of health data for a broad range of uses, including primary care decision making, public health activities, consumer education, and academic research.[16] That was another important step. But it was only a step, particularly because as originally conceived, the idea was limited to improving clinical decision making, safety, and quality. The idea has far broader applications.

The same principles are fundamental to both the Learning Healthcare System and precision community health: evidence-informed intervention that rests on analyzing, applying, and sharing a wealth of health information at many scales and with many stakeholders. This is increasingly seen as the standard way public health needs to do business, though that was not at all the case when I entered the field.

The roots of the learning approach can be seen in the ways Kaiser Permanente has applied the wealth of data it has collected over the decades. Kaiser Permanente has always been a data-driven organization, going back to when Morris Collen and his colleagues helped create the most comprehensive inpatient and outpatient medical information system in the world. Although the multiphasic exam was phased out in the 1980s, the research databases it created are still very much alive. In 2016, for example, Kaiser Permanente launched a five-year, $13 million study to revisit those exams to evaluate how risk factors in early life and midlife have affected brain health and dementia risk among a large, ethnically diverse cohort of seniors. In particular, researchers aim to explore how early-life conditions may play a role in racial and ethnic differences in dementia rates and risk factors for cognitive decline, an area that has not been well studied.

"This study is like time travel, allowing us to look at risk and protective factors for cognitive decline throughout one's life," said Rachel Whitmer, principal investigator of the new study and research scientist with the Kaiser Permanente Northern California Division of Research.

"We'll be able to analyze how factors such as midlife vascular health, psychosocial conditions, and early-life growth indicators have influenced brain health and dementia risk among current members of Kaiser Permanente."[17]

Kaiser Permanente has a long track record of applying data in clinical settings, and the systems have evolved to the point at which physicians will be able to predict which hospitalized patients are at risk of ending up in the intensive care unit. We are in the relatively early stages of exploring how the same approach translates into improving community health as well. The potential impact is already evident, however. The wealth of clinical data we have on our patients may help us, for example, find public housing for someone facing homelessness or connect an expectant mother with food aid. These kinds of interventions, preventing individual suffering before it begins, are a clear goal of precision community health.

From Public Health to Hackathons

The potential applications of new technology to public health, privacy concerns, and the principles of a Learning Healthcare System are vitally important topics, but from the perspective of a public health official, they can also be a bit abstract. One of the first projects we undertook to leverage data to improve the health of Chicagoans grew out of something far more tangible and, sadly, familiar to anyone in public service: frustration. The city's Department of Innovation and Technology (DoIT), under the leadership of John Tolva, Brett Goldstein, and Brenna Berman, had taken great strides to build a data portal and make Chicago a leader in using vast amounts of information to bring city management into the twenty-first century. From a public health perspective, we were not using all that information to tell a story that anyone other than an academic data scientist could appreciate. I wanted to aggregate that data and visualize it so we could explain the health of the city to anyone.

I contacted Daniel O'Neil, a computer scientist who had been working with the city's innovation team on software to predict hot spots of crime. Dan and some volunteer software developers then set out to build the Chicago Health Atlas, a mapping tool with information about various health conditions and access to resources online. The Atlas is designed to provide policy makers, health practitioners, and community advocates with detailed information about the health challenges of their particular communities, as well as possible solutions.

The first version of the Atlas was a simple lookup tool for existing data. From there, it expanded to include health records stripped of personal identifying information, gleaned from a variety of sources, including local hospitals, and connect them to geographic mapping points. We started with a few hundred data sets; now more than six hundred are accessible through the map interface. Today, the Atlas generates community profiles so that medical providers can understand the social, environmental, and economic context of their patients and make better clinical decisions.

The Chicago Health Atlas draws data from a diverse range of sources, including the City of Chicago data portal, CDPH programs, electronic health record data from academic health centers in Chicago, data from partners such as Purple Binder on local community and social resources, and City of Chicago web portal aggregate data. Together, these contribute to profiles that show how health outcomes, demographics, and assets intersect in each Chicago community.

The Chicago Health Atlas was built by informatics researchers at health systems, hospitals, and universities in Chicago. Since the initial formation of the partnership, the Atlas has been expanded by the Smart Chicago Collaborative—a civic organization devoted to improving lives in Chicago through technology—to include data and research from the CDPH and other agencies. The first director of the Smart Chicago Collaborative was none other than Dan O'Neil.

The Atlas was just one example of the value of public-private partnerships. The CDPH, like nearly every other public health department in the country, was strapped for cash and had little capacity in data analysis and application development. We just knew the problems that we had to solve.

That is why people like Dan O'Neil, Jay Bhatt, a geriatrician interested in innovation, and Raed Mansour, director of innovation at the CDPH, were so important. Public agencies are generally risk averse. I felt that we needed to act like entrepreneurs and bring together nontraditional partners with nontraditional skill sets to make use of new technologies. The sources of data of interest to public health grew by many orders of magnitude so quickly that we did not know how to process it all.

That realization led me down another surprising path to someplace I never imagined I'd be as a public health professional: a hackathon. These events, which became popular in the mid-2000s, bring together software developers for a period of intensive coding—anywhere from a few hours to a few days—with the goal of getting a workable product out by the end of the session. Chicago's version is called Chi Hack Night, and it has been a weekly event since 2012. The idea, which has come to be called the civic tech movement, is to bring together technology experts willing to volunteer their time and expertise to improve the lives of community members.

We were lucky in that Chicago has a long history of civic organizing as well as a more recent history of civic technology. One of the catalysts for innovation in the city is Chicago's leading tech startup center, named 1871 in honor of the Great Chicago Fire. Originally funded by a $2.3 million grant from the State of Illinois and private sponsorships, it's located in Chicago's iconic Art Deco Merchandise Mart, with the purpose of increasing innovation and job growth in the region. A hub for digital startups, the center opened its doors in 2012 with fifty thousand square feet of space for a wide variety of tech startups.

I didn't know what 1871 was, and I had only a general idea of what a tech startup was. I had no idea what to expect from Chi Hack Night, but I decided to treat it as just another opportunity for coalition building. I was used to town halls and roundtable discussions filled with activists of various descriptions. But 1871 was not the usual office and was not filled with the usual people—lots of jeans and T-shirts and piercings—and I felt like a fish out of water. But it was immediately obvious that everyone who had come that night was interested in trying to solve real problems, and the main issue would be how to harness their commitment, excitement, and talent.

It turned out not to be hard at all. I began by saying that the CDPH was looking for help in making our data available. Coders began throwing out ideas, brainstorming what might work. Among the first people to volunteer for Chi Hack Night was a web applications developer from the University of Chicago named Tom Kompare. He was interested in the free flu shot clinic locations, since flu season was coming up fast. So he went to work, and within a week he had taken a static website with the flu shot information and converted it to a web application that could be accessed on a mobile device. Within a few months, we released the flu shot app to the public. All the code was free and available to anyone, so other cities, including Boston and Philadelphia, adopted the idea too.

Then, while using Twitter in 2013, I noticed a tweet by someone who said they got sick after eating at a specific restaurant. I asked an inspector to check it out, but it also made me think we were sitting on a rich vein of data and did not even realize it. As with the Health Atlas, I wanted to take full advantage of the information that we already had. How many other people were out there tweeting about dirty restaurants but not telling the health department? I began using the social media management software Hootsuite to search for other tweets about people getting sick in Chicago after eating out. Even a rather simple search showed that, indeed, social media were full of potentially useful information, if we could capture and organize it a timely fashion.

Once again we reached out to the civic tech community for help. In few months they had an app and a website, Foodborne Chicago, that automates searching Twitter and routing the messages related to foodborne illnesses to inspectors, who follow up and encourage the Twitter user to file a complaint through the city's Open311 system. Foodborne Chicago uses a program designed to detect language that suggests an individual may be suffering from food poisoning. First, we identify the local Twitter users who have posted information suggesting that a particular restaurant has been the cause of food poisoning. Then we review the content of the tweets more closely to identify instances that are likely to represent actual foodborne illness. We then respond to residents via Twitter and ask them to file a complaint with the CDPH. The app complements the city's 311 telephone reporting system by providing an online option to report to the CDPH, and it sends the residents a form via Twitter to complete once they have reported a potential foodborne illness via tweet to Foodborne Chicago. In the first ten months after launching Foodborne Chicago, project staff identified 270 tweets with specific complaints of foodborne illness, leading to 193 complaints of food poisoning submitted to Foodborne Chicago. Ten percent of those who filed complaints sought medical care, and a total of 133 establishments received health inspections.[18]

Nearly 92 percent of those immediately targeted for inspection were cited with at least one violation. More important, 20 percent revealed at least one critical violation, or an "immediate health hazard." Critical violations are more likely to result in foodborne illness and must be fixed immediately or else the establishment gets shuttered. These examples underscore how open data, social media, and mobile technologies can be used together to monitor and protect public health.

Foodborne Chicago, the flu shot app, and the Chicago Health Atlas were all important steps because they demonstrated the power of leveraging all the data that various agencies were collecting but not using or not using effectively. We began to open the eyes of community members, partners, and politicians to the state of health in their community and to the kinds of tools we could build to improve it. Everyone was starting to understand in tangible ways the potential of big data. And it was only the beginning.

Free the Data!

Public health was just one part of Chicago's wholehearted embrace of new technology. Mayor Rahm Emanuel was committed not just to Healthy Chicago but also to Smart Chicago—a city that takes full advantage of new tools to improve the lives of its residents. That means using data technology to improve mobility, services, and infrastructure. But all of that rests on something more fundamental: making data accessible to whoever needs the data. Few phrases conjure images of dust and cobwebs more effectively than *municipal archive*, but today these archives are dynamic repositories that are ever more central to the lives of great cities, fundamental to transparency, efficiency, and innovation.

Mayor Emanuel was committed to the idea of liberating data—making as much information public as possible, within the bounds of privacy, and allowing the tech community to use the data to serve our population. Even before his inauguration, Mayor Emanuel set an ambitious agenda that specifically called for technology to lead the way for more government efficiency and transparency. Included in his goals for the new administration was a directive to use an open data model to publicize city records and to centralize many of the city's internal service operations.[19]

Chicago collects a plethora of data every day—information on everything from weather to traffic patterns to the location of libraries, schools, sidewalks, and public parks. But this abundance of data in itself can't solve urban problems. Most of the data exist in separate systems, often in conflicting and confusing formats. In effect, the data were trapped. We had to break them out of their silos so we could build tools to sift through them and offer useful insights. Only then could government managers and communities actually tap all that information to make better decisions.

Liberating data is an important component of Chicago's innovation strategy. The goal of open data is to put information that is underutilized by the government in the hands of people who can unlock its potential value. By increasing the flow of information, the open data model creates opportunities for government leaders and their teams to analyze the data to improve outcomes, look for inefficiencies, and communicate better with their constituents.

Chicago has been at the forefront of the data liberation movement in cities. The strategy involves many players, including City of Chicago departments and agencies, technology companies, entrepreneurial hubs for digital startups, and civic organizations, such as the Smart Chicago Collaborative. To begin, Mayor Emanuel asked each city agency to focus on innovation with guidance from the Digital Excellence Initiative. One of the inaugural efforts to leverage technology was the Open311 project. Open311 grew from a partnership between the mayor's office, Chicago's Department of Innovation and Technology (DoIT), and Code for America, a not-for-profit group that helps residents and governments harness technology to solve community problems. This project used phone-based technologies to foster open communication about issues related to public space and public services, making 311 calls transparent to the public. The project also included a response tracker so that residents could identify how the call was resolved.

Data liberation also spurs innovation by giving developers access to information that can be used in application development, analysis, data visualization, and so forth. Applications are often adopted by the city or by civic communities that share their knowledge to develop open-source projects for the city. Predictive analytics uses many variables that are often derived from open data sources, such as weather, 311 complaints, business licenses, and so forth.

Chicago launched its SmartData platform in 2014. SmartData gives leaders a tool to search for relevant data and detect relationships, analyzing millions of lines of data in real time. This helps city officials make smarter, speedier decisions to address a wide range of urban challenges. At its core, it makes data-driven government the norm and can fundamentally alter the way the city operates.

This project created a platform to help city employees use available data to prevent problems before they develop. The platform is connected to WindyGrid, a data hub that houses real-time information and gathers millions of data records each day from city departments.

With this kind of information, public health officials may be able to better respond to possible public health issues by, for example, providing prenatal treatments to prevent birth complications, recommending dietary changes that will help manage a chronic disease, or distributing vaccines early to contain a viral outbreak. Wise use of public health data through well-designed predictive analytics could transform how government operates and how resources are allocated.

There is a great opportunity in public health to use analytics to promote data-driven policies. We need to use our data better, share it with the public and our partners, and then leverage the data to create better policies, systems, and environmental changes.

As departments across Chicago's city government began to focus on innovative uses of data, it became increasingly clear to me that there was a need for cross-sector relationships anchored by local and state health departments. Neither health departments nor health systems can navigate this terrain alone—nor should they. Working together, these organizations—governments, health plans, academic delivery systems, community-based organizations, and the private sector—have the potential to leverage data and technology to transform public health. To evaluate the success of open data, a city can be accountable for the number of data sets, the number of applications developed, and the economic multiplier effect of small businesses created as a result of open data. Increased economic development through civic innovation is most often viewed through the lens of open data.

Predictions Are Hard, Especially about the Future

The Health Atlas and the flu app made data available in new ways and for new purposes. Smart Chicago was liberating more and more data. But I wanted to use data not just to inform people about what had happened in the past, or even what was happening right now, but what might be about to happen. That is the crux of public health: to intervene before an outbreak of disease becomes a full-on epidemic, before a neighborhood problem becomes a citywide, or even nationwide, crisis.

Consider again our work with restaurants and health code violations. Our methods were firmly rooted in New Deal–era regulations. What is known as the federal Food Code has evolved since it was introduced in 1934, but the fundamentals have remained—the familiar A, B, C cleanliness ratings you often see posted in restaurant windows. To keep Chicago's sixteen thousand food establishments safe, the city was divided into districts, each headed by a supervising sanitarian, with a team of food sanitarians who rotated across the districts and inspected every restaurant once a year or responded to reports of problems. Even the title *sanitarian* reflects the roots of urban health initiatives in nineteenth-century ideas of public hygiene. Treatment of lead toxicity was built on a similar wait-and-see approach: wait until we know that a child has poisoning, and then start treatment and send out inspectors to remediate lead in the child's home.

That system worked to a large extent and is still in place. But at the time, there were only thirty-two health inspectors for the entire city, so it is not the most efficient use of scarce resources, and it does not leverage the tools we have at hand. Most important, it is reactive—health departments close restaurants after they find violations or even after people have already become sick. We can do better.

To understand how, we need to recognize that technology has moved from the medical care system to the forefront of public health. In 2008, Dr. Donald Berwick, a founder of the Institute for Healthcare Improvement and one of the leaders in health-care reform in the United States, developed a framework for optimizing health system performance that he called the Triple Aim: improve the experience of care; improve the health of populations; and reduce the costs. Berwick went on to help implement the ACA as administrator of the Centers for Medicare and Medicaid Services, and the Triple Aim became a guidepost for a whole host of innovations to improve health. Practitioners and policy makers quickly realized that a key component would be identifying individuals at higher risk so that health-care systems could become more strategic about allocating resources. A tool called predictive analytics created opportunities for customized prediction and relative risk scores to achieve the goals of Triple Aim.

Predictive analytics describes statistical and analytical techniques to explore data—current, historical, or both—for clues about the future. A central part of the process is identifying patterns in the data and building formulas based on those patterns that health-care providers can use to more accurately identify patients in need. Without this tool, many patients who are at increased risk may be overlooked, and opportunities for prevention may be lost. By harnessing a diverse set of data sources, including homegrown, community-specific data, accurate prediction becomes plausible.

One early pilot project focused on rodent baiting and demonstrated how Chicago could use predictive analytics to improve basic city services. Rodent complaints are one of the city's top ten 311 inquiries—there were forty thousand of them in 2018. Traditionally, the city was reactive, sending out workers to bait rodents when there was a complaint or a specific event, such as a water main break, that was anecdotally linked to rodent activity.

The Smart Chicago Collaborative was again at the forefront in looking for a better way, this time analyzing three years' worth of data along with complaints about such things as overflowing trash bins, tree debris, food poisoning at restaurants, and vacant buildings. In the search for signals that precede clusters of rat complaints, data scientists fed all those data into a program to determine how accurate it was in predicting where and when populations would spike next. They found that calls related to food and shelter were the strongest predictors of a rat infestation. So, areas where residents called about sanitation violations or tree debris were most likely to see a spike in rat complaints. On the basis of historical data, the scientists were able to predict a spike in rodent complaints a full week before it happened.

Rat control was obviously a health concern, but it was not actually the responsibility of the CDPH. I was aware of this kind of work but hardly an expert in it.

Foodborne Chicago had been a big step, but I felt that we were still just scratching the surface. Tweets were obviously a rich source of data, but they were just one stream in a potentially huge river—other social media reports, building code violations, sourcing of food, registered complaints, lighting in alleys behind food establishments, nearby construction, sanitation code violations, neighborhood population density, complaint histories of other establishments with the same owner, and more. That realization was what led me to bring in the insurance data scientists from Allstate.

The CDPH and DoIT then began to work with local partners to develop an algorithm that produced a risk score for every food establishment; the higher the score, the greater the likelihood of identifying a critical violation. The first test failed, so we retooled the variables and how to weight them. In September and October 2014, we generated a list of priority inspections and compared the projected violations with what inspectors really found. The results were clear: the algorithm found violations seven and one-half days earlier, on average, than the inspectors operating as usual did.

We generated a list of the top five hundred restaurants at risk. In the first week we found so many critical violations. One fast-food restaurant on the North Side, for example, had ants on the bread racks, fruit flies in the restrooms, and houseflies everywhere else, along with rust, plumbing problems, and other violations.

To be clear, this new system did not replace the traditional system altogether. We continued to inspect every food establishment following the established schedule. Inspectors still get their assignments from a manager, for instance, but now the manager is generating schedules from the algorithm. Gerrin Cheek Butler, director of food protection at the CDPH, was a fantastic partner in developing the new tool and was key to putting it to use across the city.

Predictive analytics allowed us to concentrate our efforts on those establishments more likely to have challenges. Even more important, it proved the concept and made it clear that we could tap big data for other pressing public health concerns. Among the most troubling was, and remains, lead toxicity.

Almost all housing in Chicago was built before the nationwide ban on lead paint in the 1970s. Just inspecting two hundred thousand or so at-risk units, by one estimate, would take nearly eighty years and cost almost one hundred million dollars. And that would cover just finding the problems, not fixing them.[20] Exposure to lead can seriously affect a child's health, causing brain and neurological injury, slowed growth and development, and hearing and speech difficulties. The consequences can be seen in our schools, where exposed children may suffer from learning and behavior problems, lower IQ, attention deficit, and underperformance. Furthermore, federal funding has decreased over the past several years, meaning there is less money to pay for inspectors to go out and identify homes with lead-based paint and clear them.

In 2013, the Illinois Department of Health reported that 10,361 children in Chicago aged five or younger had blood lead levels above five micrograms per deciliter, the level the CDC considers the threshold for lead poisoning.[21] Most live in impoverished neighborhoods on the city's West and South Sides, where the paint on walls and woodwork of deteriorated apartments and homes often predates the 1978 ban on lead-based paints. In the hardest-hit neighborhoods, as many as 10 percent of children have elevated blood lead levels, compared with 3.5 percent citywide. We clearly had a serious problem and limited resources with which to address it.

What we also had, however, were several data sets from various city agencies: the addresses where children had been poisoned by lead in the past; the results of home lead inspections; and enrollment data for the Special Supplemental Nutrition Program for Women, Infants, and Children (WIC). We also had access to public databases that contain information about city housing, such as which buildings have been reported to have housing code violations.

The data were not perfect, with misspellings and typos in the names and addresses. The data were also incomplete because the city largely depends on residents to report housing violations. But they were a start: an approach to identifying high-risk areas rather than waiting for children to turn up in hospitals with dangerous levels of lead in their blood.

We turned to academic researchers, in particular a group based at the Center for Data Science and Public Policy at the University of Chicago led by Rayid Ghani, who was fresh from leading the data team for President Barack Obama's successful 2012 reelection campaign. Ghani and his researchers built a predictive model using two decades of blood lead level tests, home lead inspections, property value assessments, and census data. The model, including location data on expectant mothers and young children, identified 378 buildings where the risk was highest. Inspecting them would take just two months and would cost the city less than two hundred thousand dollars.[22] "Compared to nearly eighty years and one hundred million dollars, we are calling this a data science success story," said Andrew Reece, one of the investigators on the project.[23]

After making numerous adjustments in the weights given to various data points, the developers created a composite risk score. They brought in AllianceChicago, a network of federally qualified health centers that uses advanced health information technology to aid clinics serving vulnerable communities. The organization helped develop software that allows clinicians providing prenatal and pediatric care to access that risk score at the point of care and immediately send alerts to the City of Chicago when it surpassed a certain level. Doctors, landlords, and city agencies can also use the risk scores generated by the model to prevent lead exposure before it happens.

That is a potentially game-changing advance, and the work has won numerous national awards. Lead screening is effective, but it detects only lead already present in the blood after children have been exposed. This project is different because it allows public health officials to determine the level of risk and limit lead exposure before the kids are screened.

After building a prototype, the team tested the tool by scoring some homes and conducting inspections based on the results. The predictions were borne out; many of the houses had the lead hazards that the model had expected.

The rollout of the tool in the summer of 2018 involved four health centers. Alerts trigger a two-step inspection process. First, licensed public health lead inspectors visit the targeted homes for a visual inspection. If they see potential lead hazards, they complete a lead inspection and develop an abatement plan.

Another key element for the program was building an application program interface (API) so the tool could be linked to electronic medical records at city-approved health-care facilities. This risk-assessment tool, when accessed through a newborn's electronic health record, can alert pediatricians if their patient is at high risk of lead exposure. Those alerts, funneled to the city, will enable municipal lead inspectors to perform home inspections before the exposure occurs. This tool also creates reminders for ordering blood lead level lab tests or contacting patients for follow-up visits.

Predicting which restaurants will fail health inspections, preventing lead exposure, ensuring clean water supplies, delivering the polio vaccine: the list goes on, but the most effective public health interventions are typically preventive. We have rarely been in a position to make such predictions with any great degree of confidence, or at least not enough confidence to compel sweeping changes in laws or behavior. Even interventions such as chlorinating water and distributing vaccines are in many ways reactive. Predictive analytics offers public health officials new ways to anticipate public health challenges so that they can intervene and stop health crises before they ever begin. It also enables public health officials to concentrate their efforts, leading to better outcomes and lower costs.

This is the promise of precision community health. And it is emerging side by side with broader technological developments that are blurring the lines between the physical, digital, and biological spheres. Nanotechnology, the Internet of Things, artificial intelligence, and many other radical advances will create new opportunities and new challenges for community health around the world.

Public institutions should increasingly employ predictive analytics to protect the health of their residents. Large, complex data sets should be analyzed for patterns, especially from diverse sources and types of data, ultimately leading to significant public health action. For the profession of public health as a whole, predictive analytics is not the future; it is already here.

CHAPTER 5

Rise above the Noise

MODERN DATA ANALYSIS TECHNIQUES, SOPHISTICATED ALGORITHMS, cutting-edge communication technology—when I began my career in public health, I never imagined these all would become critical tools for designing precision community health interventions. But I am also learning how these same technologies create new space for old-fashioned yet still effective tools. Take, for example, your pets.

People love their pets, and there is a growing body of work that demonstrates the beneficial effects of owning a pet, particularly regarding mental health. So-called therapy pets are an increasingly common sight on airplanes, in offices, on college campuses. Many of these pets are bred and trained for their work, and some, such as dogs trained to detect seizures before they begin, carry out tasks that are beyond the skills of human medical professionals. Others, however, are simply loving companions. Could your dog or cat or bird or turtle be a therapy pet?

That was the seed that led to https://therapypets.love. It is part of a campaign developed by Kaiser Permanente and the Public Good Projects (PGP), a nonprofit organization focused on using modern communication technology to change behavior. The idea was to reduce the stigma associated with mental illness by encouraging people to submit photos of their pets. PGP then worked with the Kaiser Permanente mental health team to create messages of encouragement and support and provide facts about mental health.

The site has exceeded all expectations, and it is just one part of a broader effort.

Another component of the effort, LikeOneAnother, now shares more stories from individuals with mental health conditions than any other stigma reduction campaign.

Most important, PGP harnesses data from across mainstream and social media to develop historical, real-time, and predictive analytics regarding mental health stigma in the United States. For example, in a first for any behavior change campaign, the individuals highlighted in LikeOneAnother are identified exclusively from this media monitoring. This is precision marketing in action and in service to the public welfare.

Working with Kaiser Permanente's mental health experts and community health office, PGP has built the capability to report the American public's conceptualization of mental health. This reporting is providing insights into perceptions about mental health, including how narratives about mental health differ state by state, how people with schizophrenia are often referenced as being inherently dangerous, and how unintentionally stigmatizing behavior or language is more common than overtly stigmatizing behavior or messages in social and traditional media.

This kind of modern communication technology offers new tools for public health, but it creates its own challenges as well, particularly for young people. The explosion of new media and the instant availability of news, information—some of it accurate, much of it little more than gossip and innuendo—and seemingly endless chatter threatens to overwhelm messages about vital public health concerns.

If precision community health is to meet its potential, we need to find even more ways to cut through the clutter of confusing and often misleading messages. That means creating new, dramatic, and even controversial ways to reach people who are becoming increasingly skilled at tuning out what they don't want to hear. That is the aim of our work with PGP, and it was our aim in Chicago as well.

This chapter describes our efforts in Chicago to rise above the noise and reach specific audiences with information they can use to improve their health and their lives. Local governments are playing an increasing role in setting trends in this regard, and Chicago was way ahead of the conversation.

With Foodborne Chicago, we learned the powerful impact that social media, particularly Twitter, can have for the good of the residents of the city. As anyone who has spent any time at all on Twitter or Instagram or Facebook or any of the dozens of alternatives can tell you, however, not all of the power of social media is wielded for good. Sadly, the balance is likely on the other side of the ledger.

Twitter and Its Discontents

The Chicago Department of Public Health (CDPH) received an object lesson in the reality of social media's dark side in early 2014. The city council was preparing to vote on whether e-cigarettes should be regulated just like other tobacco products (see chapter 6 for a discussion of the policy and politics of such regulation). Little did we know at the time that e-cigarettes would, just a few years later, become one of the leading public health crises in the country—as even the Donald Trump administration, not known as a friend to regulation, acknowledged. We were simply trying to address the problem we saw in Chicago: it was far too easy for children to buy e-cigarettes.

A week prior to a city council vote, the CDPH launched a one-day Twitter campaign about e-cigarettes. Our Twitter campaigns were typically short, given the many other priorities of the department and the varied interests of our constituents. We used the hashtag #ECigTruths to facilitate engagement with the tweets. Hashtags (#) are metadata embedded in tweets allowing users to click on the hashtagged word and see all tweets using the same hashtag. The idea was to use the hashtags to facilitate people forming groups around specific topics. We hoped to encourage people to retweet our messages and thus multiply the reach of the CDPH many times over.

The proposed new ordinance in Chicago would have limited where people could vape their e-cigarettes. On January 8, 2014, we sent out a series of tweets, all of which were true and none of which was in any way hostile or aggressive—in fact, we directly invited engagement by ending the first e-cigarette tweet with "Let's talk about it!":

10:05am　#ECigs look like, are labeled & contain nicotine like cigarettes. They should be regulated as such. Let's talk about it! #ecigtruths

10:10am　#ECigs come in cotton candy, bubble gum & gummy bear flavors—clearly meant for children [URL] #ecigtruths

10:14am　The "water vapor" from #ECigs contains benzene, nickel, tin, arsenic, formaldehyde & acrolein #ecigtruths [URL]

10:18am　Percentage of middle school and high school students who used e-cigarettes DOUBLED from 2011 to 2012. They must be regulated. #ecigtruths

10:22am　Electronic cigarettes contain a dangerous, addictive drug & should be regulated like other nicotine products #ecigtruths

10:25am　We have a duty to protect our children from ever picking up a nicotine habit #ecigtruths [URL]

10:28am　Youth are particularly susceptible to behavioral advertising [URL] #ecigtruths

10:30am   We do not want to create a new generation of
           nicotine-addicted residents. It's time to regulate
           #ecigtruths [URL]

10:33am   In Chicago, smoking rates are lower than ever.
           Let's not reverse decades of life-saving progress
           #ecigtruths

10:38am   "9 Terribly Disturbing Things About Electronic
           Cigarettes" [URL] via @HuffPostBiz #ecigtruths

11:34am   Electronic cigs contain a dangerous, addictive drug
           & should be regulated like other nicotine products
           #ecigtruths

12:37pm   Safe? #ecigtruths [URL]

The first day of the campaign was for the most part quiet. There were roughly twenty tweets in response to our e-cigarette campaign, evenly divided between those for and against the policy proposal. Then, just after midnight, a Twitter user named Nick Green, who bills himself as a "youtube personality, entrepreneur and vape guru," tweeted the following: "We need to twitter bomb the hell out if [sic] @chiPublicHealth, spreading nothing but lies #kcavo #vaping . . . [URL]."

Twitter bombing is designed to fill Twitter feeds with a specific message in order to create the impression that there is a broad public consensus about a particular idea when no such consensus exists and, in fact, the dominant opinion may be the opposite of what the Twitter bombers want people to believe. In politics, this strategy has been called astroturfing, in which a movement that appears to be grassroots is in reality supported by a corporation, industry trade association, political interest group, or public relations firm. The tobacco industry has historically used astroturfing by working with third-party allies and including citizen-driven groups such as the smokers' rights movement to unite and oppose tobacco policies. Astroturfing through social media has been used with some success in elections for and against candidates and issues.

Green's tweet was visible to his followers—as of 2018 there were more than forty thousand of them—and Twitter users following #kcavo, #vaping, or both. The hashtag #kcavo is short for a saying among e-cigarette users, or vapers, "Keep calm and vape on." Green's Twitter profile connects to websites that link to pro-vaping advocacy groups and conferences and an e-cigarette-related business.

The Twitter bomb exploded. Over the next six days, nearly seven hundred tweets and retweets about e-cigarettes, including a mention of @ChiPublicHealth, were sent by more than three hundred Twitter users.

In order to better understand how social media were used to oppose the Chicago e-cigarette policy, we teamed up with colleagues from Washington University in St. Louis and the CDPH to examine patterns of Twitter use, connections among Twitter users, and content of tweets sent during the week between the campaign and the vote. To our knowledge, this was the first analysis of a Twitter bombing of a public health organization or topic.[1] Examining this particular Twitter bomb can help local health departments anticipate, recognize, and respond to social media attacks, as well as shed light on advertising as it relates to community health.

Nearly 90 percent of the tweets and retweets were against the e-cigarette policy. More than half of those suggested e-cigarettes help smokers quit and are healthier than cigarettes; over one-third "asserted that the health department was lying or disseminating propaganda." All told, the number of anti-policy tweets was more than ten times higher than the number of pro-policy tweets.

That was not a surprise, given that the point of the effort was to mobilize the vaping community. But it was still discouraging to check Twitter every day and see the attacks rolling in from people I assumed would be directly impacted by the new regulations that I was certain were in the best interest of community health. When we looked more closely, however, we found evidence that we were in fact reaching the people we needed to reach. A majority of Twitter users reporting a location in their profile were from states outside Illinois or from outside the United States. Most important, Twitter users located in Chicago were significantly more likely than expected to tweet in favor of the policy.

The CDPH and five opponents of the policy were central in the network of retweeting during this week. Four of the five opponents were affiliated with e-cigarette businesses or advocacy groups, which may have credibility among supporters of e-cigarette use. Safety and science tweets were retweeted more than lies and propaganda, perhaps because of the lower-quality arguments (e.g., name-calling) in the tweets containing lies and propaganda. The majority of tweets appeared to be from legitimate Twitter users who opposed the regulation of e-cigarettes and at least one advocacy group, the Consumer Advocates for Smoke-free Alternatives Association, aiming to organize policy opposition messaging. However, our results suggested that 96 of the 683 tweets (14.1 percent) sent by 73 of the 307 Twitter users (23.8 percent) were using an account or tweet strategy consistent with astroturfing. The structure of the retweeting network was also consistent with findings from a study of astroturfing in which a small number of accounts were responsible for a large proportion of retweets contributing to trending topics.

As the day for the vote approached, I was confident that we would have the support we needed, but some doubt lingered. Those doubts deepened during the city council's debate over the policy. One alderman actually argued that if we banned vaping, which produces water vapor mixed with nicotine and heavy metals, we would end up having to ban humidifiers, and restaurants would not be allowed to boil water. It was hard to imagine an elected official saying such things in earnest, and it testifies to a general lack of scientific understanding even among elected officials. More seriously, another alderman—an avowed user of e-cigarettes—argued that the ban would discourage people such as him-self who turn to e-cigarettes as a way to kick the cigarette habit.[2]

That is a serious concern. We certainly had no interest in keeping those who were trying to quit smoking from trying e-cigs, and a 2019 study suggested that e-cigarettes may in fact help some people quit.[3] But from a community health perspective, the balance of harms clearly came down on keeping young people from ever starting to smoke in the first place. Those trying to quit are motivated enough to get and smoke their e-cigarettes despite whatever relatively minor inconveniences are in their way.

In the end, the Twitter bomb failed. On January 15, 2014, the Chi-cago City Council voted overwhelmingly, 45–4, in favor of regulating e-cigarettes as tobacco products. The regulation defined e-cigarettes as tobacco products and applied Chicago's tobacco control laws to e-cigarettes (see chapter 6 for further discussion of policy and its rela-tionship to precision community health).

Chicago was part of an accelerating national trend. When the city council voted, 3 state laws and 108 local laws restricted e-cigarette use in 100 percent smoke-free venues, and nine states restricted use in other venues. By October 1, 2018, those numbers had exploded to 14 state laws and 789 local laws restricting e-cigarette use in 100 percent smoke-free venues and 15 states restricting use in other venues, according to a list maintained by the American Nonsmokers' Rights Foundation.[4] This sweeping action at the local level played a key part in stirring the Food and Drug Administration (FDA) to finally take steps of its own.

Given all that progress, you might think that our experience with the Twitter bomb in Chicago serves as little more than another anecdote in the boundless annals of the internet age. That would be a mistake. Given the widespread use of Twitter by policy makers, including the president, and the potential of grassroots efforts to influence lawmak-ing, it is increasingly important to understand how social media advo-cacy works.

Less than a year after the Chicago City Council voted to regulate e-cigarettes in the same way as all other tobacco products, California also became embroiled in the e-cigarette information wars. California's public health department launched an awareness campaign about e-cigarettes on a new website, Still Blowing Smoke.[5] But vaping advocates were not even a step behind, and at the time of California's official launch, they launched a nearly identical site with the message that public health authorities were spreading propaganda. They called it NOT Blowing Smoke.[6]

Give the vaping advocates some credit for being clever, and they are clearly well funded. NOT Blowing Smoke is built to confuse, as it borrows fonts, design elements, and imagery from the state's website. Looked at side by side, the two websites are nearly identical. But while California's site is filled with public health warnings about e-cigarettes, the pro-vaping site downplays the health concerns and says the science proving these devices are healthy is unequivocal: "Long-term e-cigarette use can decrease cigarette consumption in smokers not willing to quit," the site reads. "E-cigarettes are less addictive than tobacco cigarettes." Under the heading "Who are we?" the pro-vaping site dodges the question—with its implicit suspicion that Big Tobacco is behind the site—to state: "Who we are is less important that what we are. We are not blowing smoke." California's campaign reminds its residents that all the Big Tobacco companies also own many e-cigarette companies, while the vaping site pushes the narrative that "vaping is small business, not Big Tobacco." That may once have been true, but not anymore: for example, in December 2018, Altria, the parent company of Philip Morris, paid $12.8 billion in cash for 35 percent of the e-cigarette company Juul's capital stock.[7]

The quick, sophisticated, and completely misleading counterattack in California was all too familiar. Big Tobacco has mastered that particular dark art and has used it for years to obscure the truth about its products. For decades, cigarette companies knew their products were harmful. But they denied those hazards, paying prominent researchers and lobbyists huge sums of money to cast doubt on the mounting evidence linking smoking with cancer, heart disease, emphysema, and a host of other ills. Big Tobacco knew it would lose if the conversation focused on the health risks of using its products, so it sought, rather successfully, to turn it into a conversation about regulation and freedom of choice.

The same tactics are also being used to muddy the debate over climate change. Just as tobacco company scientists knew about the hazards of smoking long before the general public did, oil company scientists were aware decades ago that the continued use of fossil fuels could lead to devastating climate change. As with cigarettes, the public health implications are as clear as they are dire, yet public debate over both the urgency of the problem and the possible solutions has been hamstrung by well-funded but largely hidden campaigns to undermine consensus on basic scientific facts.

As with climate change, one tactic vaping advocates are using is to attack the messenger. When researchers, anti-tobacco advocates, or public health officials voice their concerns, they are often met with a combination of doubt, vitriol, and trolling. When California's health department posted information about its e-cigarette campaign on Facebook, the page was immediately bombarded with hundreds of comments. Some of the comments were abusive and threatening, while others, in a bit of social media jujitsu, tried to turn the evil reputation of Big Tobacco—which owns many vaping companies—against its opponents, falsely claiming that public health officials are in the industry's pocket.

E-cigarettes are much newer than other tobacco products, their health impact is still unclear, and the research may eventually show that vaping is a helpful harm-reduction tool. But even if the science follows a different trajectory, the situation in California and elsewhere suggests the Big Tobacco marketing playbook is being rolled out once again.

The hostilities are not just playing out on Twitter, Facebook, and internet comment sections. Big Tobacco and its supporters—official or otherwise—take the fight even into the most respected of scientific journals. The British medical journal the *Lancet*, which has been in publication since 1823, is no stranger to vigorous debate, but those debates now have a very different tenor. In 2014, one supporter of vaping wrote a letter to the journal alleging that the public health community insults and ignores the supporters of e-cigarettes. In response, four public health researchers pointed out that a *Lancet*–London School of Hygiene & Tropical Medicine Global Health Lab held in London debating the tobacco endgame, which was widely advertised, was an opportunity to engage on this issue. Rather than put forward their arguments, the researchers say, advocates of e-cigarettes instead chose to remain silent in the lecture theater while insulting the participants on Twitter. One example among many: a tweet directed at two of the four researchers who wrote to the *Lancet* contained a picture of a noose with the caption "Your days are numbered."[8]

We are clearly in a new world for community health, and we will need new social media strategies to combat novel marketing efforts and to increase the presence of public health on social media platforms. In Chicago, the number of tweets against the e-cigarette policy was more than ten times higher than the number of pro-policy tweets, despite high policy support from local tweeters. A number of Chicago aldermen called me personally and said they were getting lots of tweets against the policy, and they did not even realize they were the victims of a sophisticated astroturfing campaign. As they did offline or IRL (in real life), health advocates can learn from the strategies employed by pro-tobacco interests and adapt them to develop effective countermarketing.

Public health officials cannot ethically engage in astroturfing, but some of its tactics, such as coordinated use of specific hashtags (as done by the pro-vaping organization the Consumer Advocates for Smoke-free Alternatives Association) can be employed to elevate a public health topic. Public health officials can differentiate their messages from those of their opponents with high-quality arguments and reputable sources.

New media marketing strategies present both challenges and opportunities for public health. While evidence of social media affecting behavior is limited, research has shown some disturbing links—for example, an association between Facebook content and use of cigarettes and alcohol by teens. On the positive side, we are beginning to see success stories of effective online public health interventions. Both reinforce the importance of understanding social media engagement.[9]

The Perils of Menthol

Advertising is, of course, deeply entrenched in our culture. In fact, corporate America learned the lessons of precision long ago and is now immensely skilled at getting its products in front of the people most likely to buy them and, more important, keep buying them for a long time. The public health community has a lot of catching up to do.

The most obvious, and most troubling, example is the tobacco industry. The tobacco companies' ability to make their destructive products seem attractive would be awe-inspiring if it were not so malicious. The people of Chicago know Big Tobacco uses candy and fruit flavors to lure young people. They also know this is nothing new. After the FDA removed candy-flavored cigarettes from the market in 2009, the tobacco industry immediately created candy- and fruit-flavored cigarillos and cigars.

Big Tobacco claims it doesn't use these flavors to market to youth. But look closer and the truth is easy to see. Phillies brand Sugarillo Cigarillos are advertised with the tagline "When sweet isn't enough." Swisher International uses kid-friendly flavors such as peach, strawberry, tropical fusion, chocolate, grape, and blueberry—and they are called

Swisher Sweets! The pleasant minty taste and soothing, cooling qualities of menthol mask the harshness of tobacco smoke and reduce the irritation associated with nicotine, all of which increase the palatability of smoking, especially among new young smokers.

This kind of targeted marketing long predates electronic cigarettes and their flavors such as gummy bear, cotton candy, bubble gum, and Atomic Fireball. Among the most remarkable examples is the long-running campaign to sell—or, to put it more starkly, hook—African Americans on menthol cigarettes. The link between race and this particular tobacco product is undeniable and deeply entrenched: according to the CDC, nearly nine of every ten African American smokers between the ages of twelve and forty-nine prefer menthol cigarettes.[10] Overall, 70 percent of African American smokers smoke menthols, compared with 30 percent of white smokers.

The National Survey on Drug Use and Health found that 47.7 percent of all adolescent smokers smoke menthol cigarettes. In fact, kids aged twelve to seventeen smoked menthols at a higher rate than any other age group.[11] More than 72 percent of black adolescent smokers and about 48 percent of Hispanic and 52 percent of Asian American adolescent smokers used menthol cigarettes, while only 41 percent of white adolescent smokers used menthol. Of adolescent LGBT (lesbian, gay, bisexual, and transgender) smokers, 71 percent smoked menthols.

Fewer adults in the United States overall are smokers than at the time of the study, but smoking remains more common in lower-income, lower-education, and minority populations, and many of those smokers prefer menthol. Not only does menthol hook smokers at a young age, but the physiological properties of menthol can also undermine efforts to quit; there is a clear correlation between menthol cigarette smoking and severe nicotine dependence and addiction.[12] The appeal of menthol cigarettes to youth is particularly disturbing because nearly all adult smokers start as adolescents, and research has shown that these products commonly serve as a gateway to regular tobacco use.[13]

The prevalence of menthol smoking among African American communities is no accident; tobacco companies have specifically targeted these communities with marketing campaigns touting the pleasures of menthol cigarettes. This successful and pernicious effort to sell menthol cigarettes to the African American community has led to a continuing public health crisis that requires sweeping efforts to tear it out by the roots. That means both mobilizing public opinion, in some cases using marketing tools developed by Big Tobacco, and advancing innovative public policy. I address marketing here and policy in chapter 6.

Menthol is the most commonly used flavoring in tobacco products—it also is an additive in all tobacco products, a fact few smokers know. Derived from spearmint, menthol has a minty, fresh odor. It stimulates cold receptors and has an anesthetic effect, which combine to reduce tobacco smoke's harshness and give the smoker the sensation of deeper and cooler inhalation. Menthol also increases the absorption of nicotine. All those facts make clear why cigarette companies love menthol, and they raise significant questions about why, when Congress granted the FDA regulatory control over cigarettes in 2009, it chose to ban most flavored tobacco products—except for menthol.

Phoenix Matthews, a clinical psychologist and professor of health systems science at the College of Nursing at the University of Illinois at Chicago, who would play a central role in helping the CDPH develop a targeted anti-smoking campaign, argued that the twin actions of menthol make it especially insidious. "Some hypotheses believe there are two addictions—the addiction to the nicotine and an addiction to the menthol flavoring. A mentholated cough drop [could] become a trigger to increase smoking," Matthews said. "Studies have repeatedly shown that quit rates are much lower among menthol smokers," and black menthol smokers have a "much more difficult time quitting."[14]

Lloyd Hughes knew none of that in the early 1920s. Hughes—his friends knew him as Spud—was working as a cashier in his father's diner in the little Appalachian village of Mingo Junction, Ohio. Legend has it that his mother told Spud to inhale vapors from menthol crystals for his asthma, a homemade remedy still touted as an effective natural approach. When Spud stored his cigarettes in the same tin as his menthol crystals, he found they had a pleasing taste.

Whether the creation story is apocryphal or not, it is certain that Hughes was on to something. He began giving the cigarettes to local railroad and mill workers, and he developed a process for spraying tobacco with a solution of menthol, alcohol, and the oil of cassia, derived from the cinnamon tree. Hughes formed the Spud Cigarette Corporation in 1925 and sold his cigarettes door-to-door up and down the Ohio River Valley for a premium price: twenty cents for a pack of twenty.[15]

Hughes soon sold his stake in the company, but the new owner kept the brand name, and Spud Cigarettes went national. By 1932, the Axton-Fisher Tobacco Company had promoted Spud Cigarettes into the fifth-best-selling brand in the United States. In 1944, Philip Morris bought Axton-Fisher; the company continued to manufacture Spud cigarettes for domestic sales until 1963.

By that time, however, Spud cigarettes occupied just a tiny slice of the market. The obvious popularity of menthol cigarettes was clear from the start, and the big companies moved in quickly. The Brown & Williamson Tobacco Corporation introduced menthols as Penquin in 1931 and changed the name to Kool in 1933 but kept the penguin, whom they eventually named Willie.

From 1933 to 1956, menthol cigarettes generally and Kool particularly were seen as "throat" cigarettes, to be used when a cough or a cold prevented the use of one's regular brand. One 1937 ad had the penguin wearing a stethoscope and a head mirror and talking on the phone: "Tell him to switch to Kools and he'll be alright." The medical certificate on the wall read "Doctor Kool." The penguin was, naturally, smoking a cigarette. Later ads would show the penguin sporting a monocle and top hat as Kool targeted upscale smokers.

According to Phillip Gardiner, a research scientist at the Tobacco-Related Disease Research Program at the University of California who has closely studied the marketing of menthol, the Kool advertising of the day emphasized the supposed healthful nature of Kool with slogans such as "Keep a clear head with Kools. All the signs seem to point to a tough winter: cold, ice, chills and sniffles. Why not play it safe and smoke Kools?" and "Has a stuffed-up head killed your taste for smoking? Light a Kool. The mild menthol gives a cooling, soothing sensation . . . leaves your nose and throat feeling clean and clear." Kool was not only for the winter months but also for summer: "There is just enough menthol in Kools to soothe your throat and refresh your mouth no matter how hot the weather gets—no matter how hard and how long you smoke."[16]

Such claims prompted the federal government to step in, in the form of the Federal Trade Commission (FTC). In 1942, in one of the first of what would become a long series of cases arising out of cigarette advertising, the FTC pressed Brown & Williamson to stop making claims that Kool cigarettes, among other things, protected smokers from colds and were soothing to the throat.[17] The company entered into a stipulation that it would refrain from doing so, but Brown & Williamson and other makers of menthols nevertheless continued to promote the imaginary health benefits of menthol cigarettes.

Menthol smokes really took off in 1956, when the R. J. Reynolds Tobacco Company introduced Salem, the first filter-tipped menthol cigarette. Newport soon followed, and the entire menthol share grew from 5 percent in 1957 to 16 percent in 1963.

Today, about 30 percent of all cigarettes sold in the United States are flavored with menthol. (Oddly, only two countries in the world have higher rates of menthol cigarette use—the Philippines and Cameroon.) That near doubling of market share, says Gardiner, was largely due to the rise of Kool menthol cigarettes and that product's embrace by the African American community. Kool faded by the 1980s—driven down in part by rumors that Kool cigarettes contained fiberglass, that the *K* in Kool was emblematic of the Ku Klux Klan, and that Kool was a plot by racists to addict and kill blacks—but by then Big Tobacco had gained a foothold in the African American community that the industry would be loath to relinquish.

In 1953, Philip Morris commissioned the Roper Organization to conduct a general survey of Americans' smoking habits. The only menthol cigarette on the survey, and the only one of any importance in the early 1950s, was Kool. The Roper survey showed that only 2 percent of white Americans preferred the Kool brand. By contrast, the survey reported that 5 percent of African Americans preferred Kool. This small difference in preference was successfully parlayed by a new Brown & Williamson strategy centered on television advertising to position its menthol brand, Kool, and seize control of the new, expanding segregated urban black cigarette market.

What Gardiner calls the "African Americanization of menthol cigarettes" was built on an all-out advertising assault on the African American community using every available method and medium. Between 1963 and 1965, cigarette advertising more than tripled in the pages of *Ebony*, one of the main African American magazines, among them ads featuring celebrity African American endorsers such as Elston Howard, the all-star catcher for the New York Yankees. By 1962, *Ebony* carried twice as many cigarette ads as did *Life*. Tobacco company advertising executives knew from repeated surveys that African Americans were consistently more trusting of television and newspaper advertisements than were whites, and they exploited that to the fullest.[18]

Kool's advertising campaigns of the 1950s still emphasized the product's supposed health benefits, which had been the industry's mainstay message in the 1930s and 1940s. Surveys conducted by the tobacco industry during the 1960s attest to the fact that African Americans thought menthols were safer than regular cigarettes. In "A Pilot Look at the Attitudes of Negro Smokers toward Mentholated Cigarettes," Philip Morris reported that African Americans felt that menthols were the best to smoke with a cold, easier on the throat, and better for one's health.

Brown & Williamson also managed to associate Kool with rebellion, youth, and modern forward thinking that emerged with the civil rights and black power movements. Surveys from the 1960s and 1970s showed that Kool cigarette users were identified by their African American peers with attributes of bravery, toughness, ambition, and daring. The success bred imitators and led to ever more explicit marketing—African American male models with darker complexions and more pronounced African American features (the same was not true for African American women) to advertise their cigarettes, including menthols.[19] Afro hairstyles were used extensively by the Lorillard Tobacco Company to promote its menthol brand, Newport, and many advertising messages of the late 1960s and early 1970s drew their content from African American popular culture of the time. James Brown's recording "Papa's Got a Brand New Bag" was morphed by Lorillard into "Newport is a whole new bag of menthol smoking."

The word *cool* itself played no small part in the positioning of Kool cigarettes within the black community. Being cool in the African American lexicon was and is no small matter, said Gardiner; using Kool menthol cigarettes was thought by some to reinforce a slick and sophisticated image. The cool jazz movement, led by trumpeter Miles Davis, was seen as modern, current, fresh, avant-garde, and distinctly African American. By the 1980s, Brown & Williamson had launched the Kool Jazz Festival, followed by Parliament's World Beat concert series, Benson & Hedges's blues and jazz concerts, and Philip Morris's Superband series, all bringing leading black musical acts to African Americans while promoting mainly menthol cigarettes.

The predatory marketing of menthol to the African American community is not just a public health issue; it is also a social justice issue. Kwesi Harris, speaking at the Second Conference on Menthol Cigarettes, said that "the marketing of menthol to the African American community was not only targeted marketing, but also it was a question of environmental racism. . . . These products were marketed to the least informed about the health effects of smoking, [who] had the fewest resources with which to fight back, had the lowest amount of social support and had the least access to cessation services—this is indeed, a social justice issue."[20]

Given the overwhelming suffering caused by smoking, menthol has no redeeming value other than to make the poison go down more easily.[21] Just as Brown & Williamson used the media to create the Kool brand, the public health community needs to learn how to use the media to reveal the far more troubling side of that slick image. Fighting that image will require being just as creative and just as willing to push the envelope. In doing so in Chicago, we began to see how precision community health can play out.

Not All Media Are Social
The first thing we realized in working on an ad campaign was that with so many ways to get information, we would need something dramatic to cut through the media clutter. We would need to be as innovative and as provocative as we could without my getting fired in the process.

Brian Richardson, who was a key player in all our media efforts in Chicago and is now Midwest regional director for Lambda Legal, puts it succinctly: "There is a lot of crap out there; most public health ads that you see make your eyes glaze over." He's right: most of the ads from the CDC that we have all been seeing for thirty years, while well-intentioned and in some cases powerful, too often consist of sanitized, uninspired government-speak. They do not engage people at all. We needed to do much better if we wanted to get any attention in Chicago. We decided to create ad campaigns that were rooted in data but were still catchy enough to rise above the social media din that we all live with every day.

One ad went straight at the way tobacco companies have targeted the African American community. The ad showed a person's bare back that was about to branded with a hot iron labeled Big Tobacco. The clear analogy between Big Tobacco's tactics in promoting menthol addiction in the black community and slavery was edgy but not offensive to that community, according to the results of our focus groups. It had also been developed by an African American–owned advertising firm.

The ad, and the graphic assertion that what Big Tobacco was doing was akin to slavery, was too much for the mayor's office. We toned down the ad by removing the branding iron, but we kept the brand: the Burned campaign print ads featured close-ups of young people's faces scarred with the words *Big Tobacco*. The ad copy reads, "Tobacco companies use menthol-flavored cigarettes to get you addicted. Don't get burned."

That ad campaign did not stir up as much controversy as we thought it would and, frankly, as we had hoped it would. Given the stretched budget of the CDPH, we were hoping to generate earned media—newspaper stories, radio and television coverage—that would spread the ad's message far beyond what we could afford to purchase.

For our next campaign, we turned to research by Phoenix Matthews and colleagues that showed that African American lesbians were especially at risk of smoking and especially unlikely to quit.[22] Queer women of color are part of not one but several different populations that demonstrate higher smoking rates, lower quit rates, and disproportionate cancer-related deaths. We clearly needed to act, and act in a way that would reach that community directly, frankly, and in ways that resonated with their lived experience.[23]

No one had devised an anti-smoking campaign for that community, so we set out to do so. We developed a campaign that targeted African American lesbians in Chicago, a community with one of the highest smoking rates in the city. The smoking rate among all adults is about 21 percent; but the smoking rate among LGBT adults is estimated to be as high as 44 percent, and LGBT individuals are more likely to smoke more than one pack a day (47 percent versus 36 percent in the smoking population as a whole).[24] The factors driving LGBT disparities in tobacco use include stress due to social stigma and discrimination, peer pressure, aggressive marketing by the tobacco industry, and limited access to effective tobacco treatment. This disparity is troubling and unacceptable; and while we were committed to reducing smoking rates across the board, we decided to give special attention to those communities with increased rates.

In response, the CDPH launched Take Pride, an anti-smoking campaign that featured positive images of young LGBT women of color in healthy relationships, free of tobacco use. Before we ran any ads, we held focus groups with women of color across the city. They told us that the original ads were too explicit and encouraged us to change the locations where we placed the ads. Instead of typical billboards and bus stops, we put the ads inside clubs and bars, even in bathroom stalls.

One of the ads featured an image of two women kissing, a first for a public service ad in Chicago, and that raised some eyebrows when we placed it on the sides of city buses. But it got people talking. While flirtatious women were still sort of shocking in a public service ad, we received no negative responses from communities across the city.

Take Pride highlighted several CDPH anti-smoking resources, including the Illinois Tobacco Quitline and classes to help people quit smoking and to prevent young people from starting. We were proud to feature one of the first advertisements that portray queer women of color who are beautiful, healthy, and smoke-free. For young women who rarely get to look up and see themselves in an ad, the effect was powerful.

The Take Pride campaign was precision community health in action from start to finish. The entire campaign started with the data generated by Phoenix Matthews's research, so it had a strong evidence base at its foundation. Then, once we got that kernel, the creation and placement of the ads was driven by deeply engaged community members.

Pushing the Envelope

Another ad campaign in Chicago was more controversial and, as a result, more successful.

When I arrived at the CDPH, the teen birth rate in the city had been falling for more than a decade yet was still much higher than the national average. Over the next several years, we continued to move the needle in the right direction when it came to adolescent health, but there was more work to be done. Knowing that we still had a long way to go, we chose to be a little bit more provocative.

In the spring of 2013, we began to develop an ad campaign designed to spark conversations about parenting and, in turn, teens' behavior. Our Office of Adolescent and School Health, at the time headed by Suzanne Elder, an outstanding leader, rolled out a new teen-pregnancy prevention campaign.

We knew we had to do even more to break through the noise.

The heart of the campaign was a series of billboards that featured pictures of shirtless teenage boys. That alone may have raised some hackles, but we took another leap: we made the boys look pregnant.

We used images of typical high school boys—one had shaggy hair and a skateboard, another wore low-riding jeans and a baseball cap, a third was clad just in boxer shorts—but shot in a way that showed off their bare "pregnant" bellies. The tagline for each ad stated, "Unexpected?

Most teen pregnancies are. Avoid unplanned pregnancies and sexually transmitted infections. Use condoms. Or wait."

We also wanted to be driven by data, as we were with the Burned and Take Pride campaigns. We started with a similar process, looking at the data on teen births and the disparities among African American teens and others. We found that while teen pregnancies in Chicago had fallen by 33 percent between 2010 and 2015, the rate was still one and one-half times higher than the national average.[25]

As with the Take Pride campaign, the teen pregnancy ads were data driven and precise. We used geo-targeting to concentrate the ads around the city's several dozen schools and in areas with the highest rates of teen pregnancy. The advertisements were displayed on public transit buses, trains, platforms, and shelters in those areas, directing teens to resources about sexual health, contraception education, and relationships, as well as public health data and a clinic finder.

Many teens responded to the ads within days on the city's public health social media pages. We wanted to drive away the taboo of teen birth, and we believed, and still believe, that the more information teens receive, the more responsible choices they will make.

The ads were meant to shock—not for shock value alone but to get conversations started about teen pregnancies and how they really affect a community. We also wanted to make the case that teen parenthood is more than just a girl's responsibility; when a girl gets pregnant, she's not the only one who suffers. The daughters of teen mothers are more likely to become teen moms themselves. And the sons of teen moms are more likely to go to prison. These are challenges that go beyond one girl or one woman.

Chicago was not the first city to run such ads. In 1970, the advertising firm CramerSaatchi—which would soon be renamed Saatchi & Saatchi and become a global industry giant—was asked to develop an ad for the Family Planning Association in the United Kingdom. The goal was a poster that could hang in the waiting rooms of doctors' offices and bring attention to the importance of contraception. The agency got much more.

CramerSaatchi came up with the idea of taking an average white man of indeterminate age—he could be in his twenties or his thirties—and dressing him conservatively in a V-neck sweater, but making him appear heavily pregnant. He gazes into the camera with a mix of befuddlement and exhaustion. Below him is a simple tagline: "Would you be more careful if it was you that got pregnant?"

Although the ad, soon dubbed Pregnant Man, had limited distribution, it found its way into *Time* magazine. Soon it was the topic of numerous editorials and earned a Design and Art Direction (D&AD) award. More important, it was an early example of a viral ad, at a time when going viral was far more difficult. Images of the ad are still easy to find on the internet, nearly fifty years after it first appeared.

The ad also helped put its creative firm on the map. In the book *Saatchi & Saatchi: The Inside Story*, John Hegarty, who worked on the campaign, says: "The Pregnant Man was more than just a piece of advertising; it was the first time I had seen a piece of work that moved beyond the accepted boundaries our business operated in, commanding attention from a far wider group of people."[26] Pregnant Man will forever be associated with Saatchi & Saatchi—the agency even named its in-house pub in honor of the piece of work that did so much to establish its creative credentials.

Perhaps Pregnant Man was too far ahead of its time. No one else chose to do anything similar until 2009. At that time, Milwaukee had one of the highest rates of teen births in the nation, and rates for black teens were five times higher than for whites. Worst of all, teen pregnancy was a symptom of deeper problems: sexual abuse, incest, dating violence, and statutory rape.[27] The city launched a broad campaign to raise awareness of the issue, which included a new sex education curriculum for the public schools and an ad campaign. One advertisement said: "Your baby's not a baby anymore. Talk to your teen about sex." Other advertisements stated: "Think your teen life won't change with a baby?" Among the ads were several featuring teenage boys, shirtless and appearing pregnant. The tagline this time: "It shouldn't be any less disturbing when it's a girl."

The program worked. By 2016, Milwaukee's birth rate for teens between the ages of fifteen and seventeen had reached an all-time low. In 2015, there were 18.1 babies born for every 1,000 females aged fifteen to seventeen living in the city. That was down from 2014, when there were 23.9 newborns for every 1,000 females in the same age group, according to data from the Milwaukee Health Department. The city's teen birth rate has declined by 65 percent since 2006, compared with a 54 percent decline across the United States.[28] The firm that created the pregnant boy ads said the ads alone had led to a 10 percent reduction in teen pregnancy.

Milwaukee is less than one-quarter the size of Chicago. Its version of the teen pregnancy campaign, while successful, did not break into the national consciousness or beyond. That is what we were hoping for in Chicago, and that is what we got.

We wanted the ads to be provocative. We wanted those images to generate the kind of earned media coverage that the Burned campaign had not, and that's exactly what happened. The ads were featured on every local news channel and generated national and international news coverage—*Today*, the *Wendy Williams Show*, *Good Morning America*, *The View*, and even in Japan. The exact nature of the coverage was secondary: we would rather they talk about our ad for five minutes, not the latest from Kim Kardashian. Overall, the campaign received over one billion impressions and took on a life of its own.

This is not to say all reactions were positive. There was some resistance from the trans community to the implicit suggestion that people who identify as male cannot get pregnant. Some parents objected as well. One mother wrote in to complain that she had been on the train with her fourteen-year-old daughter, who saw the ad and asked, "'Why is that boy pregnant?' I don't want to have that conversation." To me, that was exactly what we wanted from the ads, even if the conversation might be awkward.

The online magazine *Jezebel* called the ads "weird" and referred to the campaign as the latest "Offensive But Hopefully Effective Teen Pregnancy campaign." Advertising targeted to teens in an attempt to better their behavior is notoriously heavy-handed, according to *Jezebel*, as if the only way to get through to a younger generation were to lecture without nuance but by using extreme imagery and scenarios.[29]

About the same we launched our campaign in Chicago, New York was taking its own provocative approach. New York's ad campaign, consisting of posters in bus shelters and subway stations, featured pictures of toddlers next to messages that read: "Honestly, Mom . . . Chances are he won't stay with you" and "I'm twice as likely not to graduate high school because you had me as a teen."

Those ads were accused of using threats and ridicule to "promote the difficulties of teen pregnancy" instead of offering assistance and education to address what the city's Human Resources Administration called "the real costs of teen pregnancy for teens and their children." Planned Parenthood of New York City denounced the ads, saying they are not the answer. Rather than offering alternative aspirations for young people, the organization said, the ad campaign created stigma, hostility, and negative public opinions about teen pregnancy and parenthood.

Opponents of New York's ads also said the city would have been better off spending its money helping teens access health care, birth control, and high-quality sexual and reproductive health education, not on an ad campaign intended to create shock value. But there is evidence that the ads worked. New York had a 27 percent decline in teen pregnancy rates following the campaign.

It is difficult to attribute all such declines to any particular ad or even any broad campaign. Many factors contribute to teen pregnancy, including lack of information about sexual and reproductive rights and lack of access to contraception and other health services. But the evidence that public awareness campaigns at the very least contribute to these declines seems to me to be undeniable, and everything we know about how people process such information suggests that sometimes you need to shock people to get them to pay attention.

That is why Chicago followed up the pregnant boys ads with another campaign. The sequence seemed obvious: What would happen if those pregnant boys gave birth and became dads?

The point was to remind all teens that parenting is a very "big" responsibility. Called Big Baby, the campaign featured an attention-grabbing image of a teen boy holding a giant baby, a baby even larger than the teen himself, who is noticeably weighed down by the new arrival. Below the image, the text reads "Not ready for the heavy responsibility of being a parent? Then carry something lighter. Use condoms. Or wait."

Like the pregnant boys campaign, Big Baby challenges gender stereotypes by featuring a young male parent, reminding residents that pregnancy and healthy sexual choices are not the exclusive responsibilities of teen girls. The campaign also directs youth to visit the CDPH website for information about sex, healthy relationships, condoms, and more.

Aggressive use of advertising for public health comes with its own risks, however. We knew, for example, that falling vaccination rates in some parts of the city were leading to outbreaks of preventable diseases such as measles and flu in schools. In an effort to be inclusive, we designed a billboard with a photo of a mixed-race child and the tagline "I am an outbreak." We put up several of the ads, including one on Ashland Avenue, a major north–south road, where it was visible to residents of some of the most economically challenged areas of the city.

The response was not at all what we intended. The community was angry, and people made their feelings known in the most direct way: someone painted over the words *an outbreak* and replaced them with a single word: *beautiful.* The *American Journal of Public Health* published a scathing editorial about the insensitivity of the ad, and it was correct. In our effort to reach diverse communities, we were insensitive to the fact that our ad might add to the stigma faced by minorities. Sometimes precision can come with its own set of blinders.

CHAPTER 6

Challenge the Status Quo

JUST AS WE CAN USE TECHNOLOGY and modern advertising techniques to reach people with public health messages, so too we can craft public policies to be far more precise. In fact, it will take more than billboards and ads on Pandora to meet the goals of precision community health.

Policy is the third essential ingredient of a comprehensive approach to public health, along with effective programs and creative promotion. Tobacco and related products are front and center of the public health policy debates, as they have been for many years. There is also another challenge only now getting widespread attention as a public health concern: climate change. Both are urgent, and both will require innovative policies across all levels of government.

By now the dangers of tobacco hardly need explanation, yet every day some four thousand children under the age of eighteen light their very first cigarette. Nearly one-quarter of those children will become regular smokers. They are attracted to the colorful packaging and fun flavors that hide the truth—tobacco kills.

No one working in public health can fail to see the damage that smoking does. I saw it firsthand at Crusader Community Health in Rockford, Illinois, and since, but Chicago was my first opportunity to confront the policy challenge head-on. The city was a leader in the field in many ways. In 2008, Chicago had strengthened an existing smoking ban, called the Chicago Clean Indoor Air Ordinance, so that it applied to virtually any indoor area in the city—except private homes and vehicles, designated smoking rooms at hotels, and retail tobacco shops. Smoking was also banned outdoors within fifteen feet of a building entrance.

That was an important step and in keeping with the overwhelming evidence of the dangers of secondhand smoke. In Chicago and in cities across the country, overall smoking rates are lower than ever. This progress is a direct result of lifesaving policies such as the Chicago Clean Indoor Air Ordinance. Health advocates work tirelessly to ensure we all have the right to breathe clean indoor air. Everyone should be able to expect a healthy environment when they walk into a restaurant, bar, or theater. We can't allow any regression in public health by reverting to a culture we've worked so hard to change. We need to, and can, do better for children everywhere.

As is often the case, however, good intentions were soon overrun by technology. In 2003, a Chinese pharmacist named Hon Lik patented the first version of today's standard e-cigarette: a device that uses a heating element to vaporize a flavored liquid solution that often contains nicotine. The first electronic cigarettes were designed to resemble cigarettes but emit only a vaporized liquid, not smoke, hence the term *vaping*. More recently, vaping devices have moved away from any resemblance to cigarettes and now look like flash drives. Some, in fact, can be plugged into computers just like a flash drive and recharged.

Big Tobacco, which had been searching for new and improved ways to deliver the nicotine fix for years, quickly saw its opportunity. Companies began buying up e-cigarette makers and launching their own versions.

Like menthol and other gateway products Big Tobacco has used to entice its next generation of smokers, e-cigarettes follow suit; their popularity with youth nationwide more than doubled from 2011 to 2012.

Hundreds of thousands of students have used these addictive products within a few years of their becoming widely available in the United States, around 2008. Electronic cigarettes now come in dozens of flavors, including passion fruit, cotton candy, bubble gum, gummy bear, Atomic Fireball, and orange cream soda. These kid-friendly flavors are an enticing "starter" for youth and nonsmokers, increasing nicotine addiction and frequently leading to use of combustible cigarettes.

This meteoric rise in popularity among youth was the main reason that Mayor Rahm Emanuel decided to broaden the anti-smoking ordinance again, this time to regulate e-cigarettes as tobacco products. One of Mayor Emanuel's top public health priorities was to reduce tobacco use among the young. The natural target was flavored tobacco products, including those containing the industry's most popular flavor—menthol—which, as we have seen, has a deeply racist history. Mayor Emanuel and the Chicago City Council made it clear: Big Tobacco does not belong in school zones. The e-cigarette proposal would make Chicago the second major city to ban e-cigarettes from being smoked in most public places; New York City had added e-cigarettes to its public smoking ban a month earlier, in December 2013. No one had taken on menthol the way we intended to.

To me, this issue was clear. Menthol is aimed at the African American community and at youth. E-cigarettes are an almost perfectly designed nicotine delivery system for hooking people when they are young, creating customers for life. We had to take on both scourges if we were to begin rooting smoking out of our culture.

Tackling Tobacco

The Take Pride and Burned media campaigns raised awareness of how tobacco companies were targeting particular communities in Chicago, but if we were going to make a lasting difference, we would need to change policy too. In 2009, Congress passed the Family Smoking Prevention and Tobacco Control Act, granting the Food and Drug Administration (FDA) regulatory authority over tobacco products. Emanuel, then a congressman representing Illinois's Fifth Congressional District, was a cosponsor, and the law was signed by President Barack Obama while Emanuel served as White House chief of staff. The bill gave the FDA authority to ban flavored cigarettes.

The act prohibited fruit- and candy-like additives as "characterizing flavors" in cigarettes because they have been used by tobacco companies to market specifically to youth. The law did not address e-cigarettes, as they were still largely unknown in much of the country. But e-cigarettes are labeled and marketed like cigarettes. They contain nicotine like cigarettes. They should be regulated like cigarettes.

Simply put, kids should not have easy access to e-cigarettes. Nicotine affects brain development, which continues until age twenty-five or so. Yet when we began the effort to regulate e-cigarettes in Chicago, a fourteen-year-old could walk into a store and purchase them, no questions asked. This was unacceptable. The city needed to require retailers to have a tobacco retail license in order to sell e-cigarettes, which would place these products behind the counter with the other tobacco products and out of arm's reach of our children. The government has a duty to protect children from ever picking up a nicotine habit. The preventive action Mayor Emanuel wanted to take was a long-term investment in the health and well-being of Chicago's youth.

I believed then, as I do now, that e-cigarettes are a public health menace and need the strictest regulation. According to the Centers for Disease Control and Prevention (CDC), the use of e-cigarettes among high school students increased by nearly 80 percent in 2017–2018 alone; there are now more than 3 million students using e-cigarettes.[1] Sales of e-cigarettes made by one manufacturer, Juul Labs, increased by 641 percent—from 2.2 million devices sold in 2016 to 16.2 million devices sold in 2017. By December 2017, Juul's sales accounted for nearly one in every three e-cigarette sales nationally, giving it the largest market share in the United States, and Juul products have among the highest nicotine content of any e-cigarette on the US market.[2] The company has already reached an exalted cultural status afforded few others; it has become a verb. Juuling is the hip thing for teenagers.

Another study released at the end of 2018 showed that the problem was, if anything, even more urgent. Increases in adolescent vaping from 2017 to 2018 were the largest ever recorded in the past forty-three years for any substance use by adolescents in the United States. The percentage of twelfth-grade students who reported vaping nicotine in the past thirty days nearly doubled, rising from 11 percent to 21 percent. This ten percentage point increase is twice as large as the previous record for largest-ever increase among past-thirty-day outcomes in twelfth grade. As a result of the increase, one in five twelfth-grade students vaped nicotine in the past thirty days in 2018. For secondary students in grades nine through twelve, the increases in nicotine vaping translate into at least 1.3 million additional nicotine vapers in 2018 as compared with 2017.

These results come from the University of Michigan's annual Monitoring the Future survey, which has tracked substance use among US adolescents every year since 1975 for twelfth-grade students and since 1991 for eighth- and tenth-grade students. To put the nicotine vaping increase in context, it is the largest out of more than one thousand reported year-to-year changes since 1975 for use of substances within the thirty days prior to the survey among twelfth-grade students.[3]

With the boom in users obviously comes booming revenue. According to a February 2019 analysis by Wells Fargo, the American vaporizer market would be more than $10 billion in 2020, an increase of more than 25 percent from 2017.[4] That's just a fraction of what old-fashioned smoking brings in—the US cigarette market is worth $120 billion—but cigarettes were at last showing signs that they could be on the way out.

Young people in particular were shunning them. E-cigarettes and vaping may change that if we do not move fast.

The release of the CDC data in the fall of 2018 finally spurred the FDA to act, and it began the process of limiting sales of e-cigarettes to youths. That is another important and welcome step, even if action at the federal level has been slow compared with that in cities and states. The FDA is slow to act by design because nationwide changes demand due consideration, and even if the FDA moves, the tobacco industry will use all its legal methods to slow it down—we have seen this pattern play out time and again. States are almost as slow to act, so policy making driven by mayors and local public health departments is imperative. The fact is that your mayor and city council have as much to do with your health as your physician.

Some might argue that e-cigarettes should not be regulated at all because they are safer than regular cigarettes and are intended to help people switch from more dangerous combustible cigarettes. At one time, Walgreens and CVS Pharmacy outlets in Chicago sold them as tobacco cessation products. That was close to making a false medical claim that these products are safe.

I had to send a letter to CVS and Walgreens to force them to stop selling e-cigarettes that way, but the pitch is visible everywhere. Juul, for one, has an aggressive marketing campaign pitching its products as a way to help smokers quit. If that sounds reminiscent of the early ads for menthol-flavored cigarettes saying in effect that they were good for you, that is no accident. But the logical end point for such a campaign would be for smokers to switch to e-cigarettes and then quit nicotine altogether. So, Juul and others would be selling a product that would eventually eliminate its own market. Ask yourself if you think that's likely, especially coming from an industry that has succeeded so spectacularly over the years knowing full well that it was killing its customers. Those ads are aimed not so much at adult smokers looking to quit, few of whom even know of the existence of Juul, but at political leaders. No wonder that those ads run most prominently and most frequently in the pages of the *Washington Post*.

While e-cigarettes may be safer than regular cigarettes, they have not been proven to be safe. The truth is that e-cigarette companies have not provided any scientific studies or toxicity analysis to the FDA to show that e-cigarettes pose any reduced health risk over conventional cigarettes. Laboratory tests have found that the so-called water vapor from some e-cigarettes can contain nicotine and volatile organic compounds such as benzene and toluene, heavy metals such as nickel and arsenic, and carbon compounds such as formaldehyde and acrolein, in addition to tobacco-specific nitrosamines, one of the most important groups of carcinogens in tobacco products.

Moreover, while the FDA crackdown will likely impact sales and marketing of e-cigarettes, there are as yet no federal regulations on what goes into e-cigarettes, which means that there currently are no restrictions on ingredients manufacturers can or cannot use and no restrictions on the kinds of chemicals they can emit into the indoor environment. Until more is known about these products, limiting their sale and their use in indoor areas is just good common sense.

I am also concerned that widespread use of e-cigarettes is renormalizing smoking in our society. E-cigarettes intentionally were developed to mimic the act of smoking. This distorted reinforcement of smoking as cool and acceptable sends the wrong message to our youth and undermines the existing smoking bans put in place to protect the health of the public.

The FDA's initial failure to regulate e-cigarettes was understandable. Another failure, however, was far less so. The Family Smoking Prevention and Tobacco Control Act carved a single but crucial exception. Congress deferred action on the most popular of all flavors—menthol—and instead directed the FDA to establish the Tobacco Products Scientific

Advisory Committee, consisting of leading scientific experts, to determine whether allowing menthol cigarettes was "appropriate for public health." In 2011, after an exhaustive review of the scientific evidence, this FDA-appointed committee issued a report detailing its findings on menthol cigarettes and concluding that the "removal of menthol cigarettes from the marketplace would benefit public health in the United States."[5]

Mayor Emanuel had made it clear that he wanted to move as aggressively as possible to curb smoking in Chicago, particularly among young people, and he looked to the Chicago Department of Public Health (CDPH) to come up with options. For inspiration, we looked, as Chicagoans have done for more than a century, to the words attributed to architect Daniel Burnham, who oversaw both the construction of the 1893 World's Columbian Exhibition and the rebuilding of the city after the Great Chicago Fire: "Make no little plans; they have no magic to stir men's blood and probably themselves will not be realized. Make big plans; aim high in hope and work, remembering that a noble, logical diagram once recorded will never die, but long after we are gone will be a living thing, asserting itself with ever-growing insistency."

The question we asked was simple: If we could wave our magic wand, make some bold moves, what would they be? The list was long: funding for cessation programs, age and pricing minimums for tobacco products, restriction on sales and marketing, and so on. We wanted not to nibble around the edges of the problem but rather to tackle it with a systems thinking approach. We were, however, well aware that no jurisdiction at any level—city, county, state, or national—had sought any restrictions on menthol. We knew, as did Mayor Emanuel, that there would be legal, political, and administrative challenges to whatever we decided to do.

In addition to advance planning, we were waiting for the moment at which a window of opportunity for change would open. That moment finally came on July 23, 2013, after more than a year of debate within the CDPH and more than two years after receiving the committee's report, when the FDA released its "Preliminary Scientific Evaluation of the Possible Public Health Effects of Menthol versus Nonmenthol Cigarettes." Mayor Emanuel pounced. Less than forty-eight hours later, the mayor directed the Chicago Board of Health and the CDPH to identify "winnable" policy solutions to curb the use of flavored tobacco products among the city's youth. The mayor asked the board to engage in a community-driven initiative to address this problem.

It was clear that the FDA would eventually issue regulations regarding ingredients and marketing—but local governments always have a role in regulating tobacco products. This was an issue where Chicago could lead.

Because menthol-flavored tobacco products are used so heavily by—and have a particularly devastating impact on—youth, African Americans, and the LGBT (lesbian, gay, bisexual, and transgender) community, it is critical to engage these groups in developing policy initiatives. Focusing on the importance of public health and social justice was critical to the success of Chicago's sales restriction of flavored tobacco products.

The CDPH held four town hall meetings across the city in neighborhoods with large African American, Latino, and LGBT populations on the North, South, and West Sides. Hundreds of Chicago residents attended—young and old, smokers and nonsmokers, health-care clinicians, hospital staff, social service providers, leaders in the faith community, and elected officials. We worked with traditional and nontraditional partners, not just the American Cancer Society and the American Lung Association but also others that were new to tobacco control, such as the Coalition for Asian Substance Abuse Prevention, the Chicago Hispanic Health Coalition, and the LGBT Advisory Council. Tobacco retailers and industry representatives participated in these town hall meetings, as did public health organizations and other interest groups.[6]

The first goal of the town halls was to simply listen to what people had to say about tobacco and what they favored in terms of policy changes. We heard firsthand stories of how menthol-flavored cigarettes have hurt Chicago's youth for generations. Public health professionals shared information with these stakeholders about the disparate health impact of menthol tobacco products on the local community, and many speakers described the problem of menthol products as not just a public health concern but also a social justice issue. They pointed out that years after flavored cigarettes were removed from the market, the tobacco industry continued to aggressively market menthol cigarettes and other flavored tobacco products to youth in minority communities. They noted that the tobacco industry targets those individuals least likely to have health insurance, seek medical care, or have coverage for tobacco cessation products—all of which is likely to make them lifelong smokers.

We also wanted to educate the community on the issues around tobacco, especially menthol.

The tobacco industry did not make that easy. Despite the fact that the town halls were mostly organized by leaders of the African American community, Big Tobacco accused us of criminalizing tobacco use among black kids and promoting a racist policy that targeted only the kinds of cigarettes that the black community preferred, not the white community.

There were also signs that an astroturfing campaign was under way at the town halls. At each meeting there would be a relatively small number of people each holding a four-by-six-inch card. When they got up to speak they would read from the card, and each had the same message: they claimed that they were not speaking for any one group, that it was unfair to pick on the one product that the black community uses most, and that there should be no ban on menthol. Their claims to the contrary notwithstanding, many believed those speakers had been given talking points by the National Association of Tobacco Outlets, the trade association for tobacco retailers.

The constant emphasis on opposing a ban on menthol was both curious and counterproductive. Such a ban was, in fact, never an option we considered. We knew the opposition would be fierce, so we looked for other policies and programs from the outset. But as the other side kept hammering on a ban that no one was considering, it gave policy makers the idea that as long as they did not enact an outright ban on menthol, they would be fine. Big Tobacco's strategy actually softened the ground for policy making.

Despite the organized opposition, the results of the town halls were dramatic. At Chicago State University, a public institution on the South Side with a largely African American student body, all those attending the meeting received an electronic device that allowed them to register their opinions on particular questions. At the beginning of the meeting they were asked about a policy to restrict menthol, and over half said they would oppose it. But when they were asked the same question at the end of the meeting, almost 90 percent said they would now support a restriction on menthol.

On the basis of what we heard at the town halls, we developed a comprehensive menthol report with numerous recommendations on steps that Chicago could take on its own. The four key recommendations were (1) prohibit menthol sales near schools; (2) increase cigarette taxes by 75¢ per pack; (3) create public service advertising that targets black youth; and (4) regulate electronic cigarettes in the same way as other tobacco products and raise the minimum age for buying, first to eighteen and eventually to twenty-one.

The focus on restrictions on the retail sale of certain tobacco products, rather than on their possession or use, was key and was a direct result of listening to the community. The community made it clear, and we agreed, that possession and use are not a crime. Most states have laws that prohibit the purchase, use, or possession of tobacco products by underage persons—so-called PUP laws—but penalizing children has not been proven to be an effective strategy for reducing youth smoking, and PUP laws could actually detract from more effective enforcement measures and tobacco control efforts.[7] Tobacco companies and their allies in fact have a history of supporting PUP laws as alternatives to other laws that would produce greater declines in youth smoking, such as increasing the price of cigarettes.[8]

Chicago's focus on retailers near schools was also seen as an opportunity to reduce tobacco-related health disparities. The rationale behind the city's decision to restrict sales of flavored tobacco products around schools was fairly simple. The city was aware that the tobacco industry has historically targeted certain neighborhoods for heavy advertising and retail outlets. Not only do retail outlets near schools typically contain more cigarette advertising than outlets farther from schools, but these stores are also especially common in urban minority communities.

Studies have shown that the number of tobacco retailers around schools has a significant impact on the number of kids who smoke. In fact, after controlling for census tract–derived school neighborhood characteristics, researchers found that the density of tobacco retailers in the Chicago area correlated with students' reported tobacco use. Youth smoking has increased by as much as 3.2 percent in neighborhoods with five or more tobacco retail outlets within walking distance (one-half mile) of a high school, compared with neighborhoods with no nearby tobacco retailers.

Moreover, restrictions on sales of tobacco products in other jurisdictions have successfully reduced use. In New York City, for example, the national law prohibiting the sale of flavored cigarettes and the city's law prohibiting the sale of flavored tobacco products, excluding menthol products and with the exception of retail tobacco stores, have been shown to significantly reduce flavored tobacco product sales. As a result, Chicago's proposed ordinance was a unique opportunity to curb tobacco sales in prime areas where youth were most commonly targeted.

Tax increases are rarely popular with the general public, but we had a simple rule: you can never raise cigarette taxes enough. This is not simply a matter of raising taxes for the sake of raising taxes. Raising the price of cigarettes impacts those who are the most price-sensitive consumers: children and adolescents, the groups that need the greatest deterrent to picking up that first cigarette.

I told the aldermen on the city council that a cigarette tax hike of 75¢ per pack would save lives, save health-care dollars in the long run, and add revenue. Our estimates were that the tax alone would save 3,500 lives in the long term from premature death related to tobacco, and that over 5,500 adults would quit smoking because of this tax. The tax would deter smoking even more in low-income neighborhoods.

Still, some aldermen were leery of hiking cigarette taxes, worrying that smokers would take their business to the suburbs or Indiana. In the end, they decided to raise the tax by 50¢ instead of 75¢ per pack, but it was still a major victory. I am proud to say that today Chicago has the highest cigarette tax anywhere. A pack of cigarettes in Chicago costs $12.00, over $7.00 of which goes back to the city and the state in the form of taxes, with an additional $1.01 in federal tax.

On November 26, 2013, the mayor introduced the tobacco regulations, including the tax increase and the products sales ordinance. The full city council passed it on December 11 by a vote of 48 to 2, making Chicago the first city in the United States to restrict the sale of all flavored tobacco products, including menthol. The ordinance restricted the sale of menthol-flavored cigarettes and other flavored tobacco products within five hundred feet (about two city blocks) of any school located in Chicago, with the exception of retail tobacco stores dedicated primarily to the sale of tobacco.

The new ordinance had teeth. Retailers who knowingly or repeatedly violated any provision of the ordinance could have their license revoked or suspended. That was not limited to retail tobacco licenses but applied to any and all licenses issued by any officer, department, or agency of the City of Chicago required for retail or other business operations. Violation of the ordinance would also result in a fine of $100–$400, for up to $1,000, for anyone found to have more than two offenses within a two-year period.

The city council ended up adopting these tobacco control policies by wide margins but not without vigorous debate. Opposition to the e-cigarette restrictions was stiffest, and as a result the vote on that aspect of the ordinance was tabled temporarily—that was the piece that prompted the Twitter bomb when it finally came up for a vote in January 2014 (see chapter 5).

The proposal to prohibit the sale of flavored tobacco products within five hundred feet of schools was also opposed—primarily by tobacco retailers. The ordinance affects approximately 377 of the city's 2,549 licensed tobacco retailers. Some retailers argued that including menthol-flavored tobacco products was unnecessary because menthol cigarettes are subject to the same regulations as all cigarettes and because, in their view, "menthol use in minority groups and among youth is due to enabling adults who buy cigarettes legally and provide them to minors, as well as a black market fueled by high taxes on tobacco at the city, county, state and federal level."[9]

Implementing the law proved to be a challenge. In order to identify which products were subject to the ordinance, for example, we needed to comb through nearly twelve thousand tobacco products on the market to draw up a list of restricted flavored tobacco products. But it is a never-ending process, as the market changes constantly. The CDPH continues to search wholesaler and manufacturer websites and industry newsletters, regularly adding hundreds of new products to the list.

The battle between big cities and the big tobacco companies and e-cigarette distributors is far from over. In fact, if Chicago's experience is any indication, the battle has intensified. Chicago's Department of Business Affairs and Consumer Protection believed, in the fall of 2018, that eight online retailers of vaping liquids that can be used in e-cigarette devices were selling to underage individuals in clear violation of the city ordinances. So the department launched a sting operation and found that of the forty online e-cigarette retailers, eight processed an order for e-cigarettes, accepted payment, and delivered the product but never checked the age of the buyer. In November 2018, city attorneys filed a lawsuit against the companies.

Despite all of Chicago's efforts, it is still too easy for youth to get their hands on e-cigarettes and vaping materials as well as flavored cigarettes. This is not a reflection on the policies we enacted but rather on the difficulty of the task that remains. Chicago has established itself as a national leader in tobacco control. The public health community across the United States is watching as these policies are implemented and enforced.

Some state and local governments, emboldened by Chicago's experience, are adopting similar measures or other innovative strategies to regulate menthol-flavored tobacco products. The first evidence that regulation works is coming from the province of Ontario, Canada, which implemented a full ban on menthol on January 1, 2017, and conducted a robust before-and-after study in conjunction with the new law. People said before the ban was implemented that they would continue smoking, but once menthol was banned, they decided to quit instead.[10]

We are seeing encouraging moves toward sharing information across jurisdictions on menthol and e-cigarettes. In Chicago, we worked closely with health officials in New York, San Francisco, Los Angeles, and Long Beach, and in April 2014 there was a flurry of new e-cigarette laws. This kind of collaborative effort will be vital to stemming the tide of vaping, particularly among young people.

Climate Change and Community Health

Tobacco smoke, whether from cigarettes or e-cigarettes, is a kind of air pollution and hence an environmental as well as a public health challenge.

The links between the environment and community health are becoming increasingly clear, as I saw firsthand when I traveled to Puerto Rico not long after Hurricane Maria devastated the island in 2017. Nearly three thousand people are estimated to have died as a result of the hurricane, and Puerto Rico went nearly a year without power being fully restored. That experience brought home the fact that climate change is not just an ecological or conservation problem; it is a public health crisis.

As I visited clinics around Puerto Rico, I saw the devastating, polarizing effects of climate change and its impact on vulnerable communities. Women from poorer neighborhoods told me stories about how they tried to survive without electricity and clean water. I met a man with diabetes who didn't know how to keep his insulin refrigerated and as a result his diabetes got out of control. One child told me that she worried about whether it was safe to sleep at night because another hurricane might hit her home. I also visited Puerto Rico's Department of Health and saw the complete devastation of its laboratories. These are the labs that carry out vital functions such as monitoring the safety of drinking water, analyzing blood samples, and so on.

The same dynamics were at play in Houston, Texas, when flooding during Hurricane Harvey disproportionately impacted the city's low-lying, poorer neighborhoods. Climate change is a global problem with local effects. With climate change, as we have seen with other public health challenges, your zip code is a better predictor of health outcomes than your genetic code. This explains why people in different neighborhoods can have dramatically different life expectancies. Warmer temperatures, droughts, more powerful storms, rising seas, air pollution, the condition of our homes—or whether we have homes at all—where we get our food, where our children play: these are all parts of the environment around us, and they have profound effects on our health.

Contrary to popular belief, the root causes of poor health are rarely caused only by poor individual choices. Food access is a clear example of how the environment around us affects health. A family living in poverty in a food desert may face a difficult commute to get to a full-service grocery store and instead rely on the nearest convenience store. But there, energy drinks, alcohol, tobacco products, and candy occupy most of the shelves, and frozen foods—high in sodium and saturated fat—often are the only practical dinner options. Dairy products typically are available in food deserts, but families with limited purchasing power often stretch their grocery dollars by buying cheap soda instead of the more expensive milk.

The links between an individual's environment and health have been attracting increasing attention for a decade or more. In Chicago these issues were clearest in the context of lead poisoning in low-income housing, which was one important reason the CDPH took over the permitting and enforcement functions of the city's environment department in 2011. "Upstream" efforts such as the one in Chicago seek to change systems, laws, and physical landscapes to improve health.

The broader global environment has gotten short shrift in public health circles. But that may be changing. In late 2018, the *Lancet* published "The *Lancet* Countdown on Health and Climate Change: From 25 Years of Inaction to a Global Transformation for Public Health." This independent assessment noted that the effects of climate change—rising temperatures, increasing weather-related disasters, the spread of vector-borne disease—are "potentially irreversible."[11] As the report details, the health consequences are numerous, varied, and happening now. Rising temperatures and changing precipitation patterns affect the air we breathe, contributing to respiratory and cardiovascular illnesses such as asthma and lung cancer. Worsening heat events mean more incidents of heat stroke, dehydration, nausea, and even death.

Heat not only affects us directly but also affects the creatures (vectors) that carry Lyme disease, malaria, Zika virus, West Nile virus, and other life-threatening diseases. Organisms such as ticks, mosquitoes, lice, and snails will become more widespread as the warmer climate allows them to spread into previously uninhabitable areas.

The frequency of natural disasters is also increasing as a result of extreme weather patterns. Floods, hurricanes, blizzards, and wildfires endanger lives, and their aftereffects cause both physical and mental trauma. Devastating fires may be the most obvious consequence of a hotter, drier climate, but there are others. In late 2015, California was in the fourth year of its most severe drought since becoming a state in 1850. According to the Fourth National Climate Assessment, households in drought-stricken Tulare and Mariposa Counties reported a range of health problems, including allergies and asthma from dust, not to mention acute stress. These problems were not evenly distributed, with families suffering more when drought damaged their household property and finances.

Drought can be as serious a problem as heat itself. Dry conditions increase reproduction of a fungus found in soils, potentially leading to the disease coccidioidomycosis, or valley fever. Coccidioidomycosis feels like a bad case of flu, sending its victims to the hospital and reducing workers' productivity. Cases in Arizona and California are rising as soils dry out. Through a complex series of interactions, drought can also lead to financial hardship, in turn increasing mood disorders, domestic violence, and suicide.[12]

In fact, changing weather patterns trigger a host of other dangerous changes. If farmers experience a bad growing season, it can lead to food shortages. Hotter temperatures increase the risk of salmonella poisoning, while warming waters alter the location and timing of bacterial infections in seafood, leading to gastrointestinal illnesses. Even basic access to potable water is a growing concern across the globe.

Climate change is already causing people to move as their communities become uninhabitable from rising seas, droughts, and extreme weather events. This displacement can result in mental anguish and exacerbate violence, especially in politically unstable areas. Indeed, coping with any of these effects of climate change can create and exacerbate stress.

The impact of climate change on mental health is often overlooked, but the ripple effect of severe weather events is significant for individuals and communities. Survivors of these events may experience significant emotional trauma from the event itself, as well as from losing a loved one, home, crops, or valued possessions. Additionally, some studies show suicide rates increase with temperatures, with contributing factors cited as the heat itself, loss of crops, and forced migration.[13]

The more we study the complex interactions between climate and health, the more risks we find. Rising carbon dioxide concentrations, for example, have adverse effects on the nutritional quality of major cereal crops, such as rice and wheat, including lowering the levels of protein, a range of micronutrients, and B vitamins. Climate and other environmental changes also reduce the yield of vegetables and legumes overall, which has important implications for the prevention of noncommunicable diseases.[14]

The World Health Organization (WHO) estimates that approximately 250,000 deaths annually between 2030 and 2050 could result from climate change–related increases in heat exposure in elderly people, as well as increases in diarrheal disease, malaria, dengue, coastal flooding, and childhood stunting. This is a conservative estimate because it does not include deaths from other health problems affected by climate and does not include morbidity or the effects associated with the disruption of health services from extreme weather.

The WHO estimates that climate change–related health-care costs could balloon to four billion dollars in 2030. And what about the human cost? We cannot wait idly to find out. Current warming trends are "threatening all aspects of the society in which we live, and the continuing delay in addressing the scale of the challenge increases the risks to human lives and health," the report states, stressing that "climate change is the greatest health challenge of the 21st century."[15]

So who carries the burden? Natural disasters have a disproportionate effect on the young, the elderly, and those living in poverty. In these communities, where resources and infrastructure are already strained, the ability to evacuate, receive emergency care, and find stable housing in an emergency are severely limited. With Hurricane Katrina, which hit New Orleans in 2005, we learned that inequalities—defined by income, race, and education—made people more vulnerable because of where they lived and their ability to evacuate.

The deadly and unprecedented wildfires in California in the fall of 2018 put the profound impacts of climate change on health into stark relief. The fires and the mudslides that followed destroyed thousands of homes, largely wiping out entire towns. Many residents who lost their homes will not be able to rebuild, and there are doubts that levels of affordable housing will recover.

There can be no clearer link between climate and health, because housing *is* health. Better health begins where health starts, in our communities. Health cannot happen within the walls of a doctor's office if people don't have a safe place to call home, and climate change is only making that problem even harder to solve. Not only does climate change disproportionately impact the most vulnerable communities; it is also part of a vicious cycle: climate change makes the poor poorer, and poverty impacts health, and poor health leads to even greater poverty. The World Bank estimates that without climate-resilient development (i.e., development that helps communities to absorb climate shocks and create coping strategies), climate change could force more than one hundred million people into extreme poverty by 2030.[16]

Natural disasters such as fires and hurricanes do not affect only those directly in their path. After people with resources flee from the danger zone or seek medical help, those left behind must deal with the ongoing crisis. Eventually, as the effects of climate change spread across regions and communities, we will all feel its impacts, and humanity as a whole will pay the price. That is why we all have a role to play—and a responsibility to act.

At the most basic level, the public health community can contribute by providing affordable, quality health care for people harmed by climate change. But we also have to expand our vision of public health by thinking systemically when it comes to climate change. Health advocates should embrace strategies for combating climate change with the same vigor that they now endorse smoking bans or lead abatement.

Shifting from fossil fuels to renewable power creates immediate public health benefits because it reduces air pollution, and that lowers the risk for asthma and other respiratory diseases. Walking, cycling, and taking transit instead of driving reduces chronic diseases and air pollution.

Climate-Smart Health Care

The public health community has a central and multifaceted role to play in responding to climate change. First and foremost, we are health providers. Hospitals, health centers, emergency medical technicians, nurses, and doctors are on the front lines when a hurricane or wildfire hits. We must have resilient infrastructure that remains operational even during the most extreme weather events. Health-care systems must also prepare for longer-term climate-induced changes in disease patterns.

Although health-care systems are crucial to treating the effects of climate change, they are also contributing to the problem itself. Health-care activities account for up to 10 percent of greenhouse gas emissions in the United States. Fortunately, forward-looking leaders in health care have started lowering their institutions' carbon footprints and becoming more energy efficient.

In 2017 the World Bank published a report, coproduced with the nonprofit organization Health Care Without Harm, that lays out how a low-carbon approach can provide effective, cheaper care while at the same time being "climate smart."[17] That means designing, building, operating, and investing in health systems and facilities that generate minimal amounts of greenhouse gases. Climate-smart health care not only saves money by reducing energy and resource costs; it also helps ensure that key facilities will be able to withstand the climate-induced disasters we know are coming.

In June 2018, the Health Care Climate Challenge was launched to mobilize health-care institutions around the world. Thousands of hospitals, health centers, and entire health systems are already implementing climate-smart strategies. I'm proud to work for one of the leaders.

When Kaiser Permanente's environmental work began twenty years ago, the focus was on getting mercury and hazardous materials out of supplies and building materials. More recently, Kaiser Permanente called on suppliers to eliminate toxic flame retardants and introduced safer cleaning systems to protect patients and workers. Today, we look across the entire health-care sector and ask how we can reduce our considerable environmental footprint. That kind of systemic thinking has created a powerful vision for us as an organization.

We understand that climate change threatens health, and our work to mitigate that damage is embedded in our operations—in how we manage buildings, purchase food, medical supplies, and equipment, and serve our members, as well as how we consume energy and process waste. Kaiser Permanente was the first health-care organization in the nation to begin monitoring and publicly reporting our greenhouse gas emissions, beginning in our California regions in 2005. We now track greenhouse gas emissions across our operations. In September 2018, we announced a major renewable energy purchase that will allow us to reach our goal of being carbon neutral in 2020.

Our 2025 Environmental Stewardship Goals are designed to further reduce our climate footprint. Among these steps are to become carbon net positive by removing more greenhouse gases from the atmosphere than we emit; to reduce, recycle, or reuse 100 percent of our nonhazardous waste; and to buy all of our food locally or from producers that use sustainable practices, including using antibiotics responsibly. And we will do this even as we anticipate that our organization will continue to grow.

By reducing emissions in our own institutions and throughout our supply chains, health-care organizations can be catalysts for decarbonization across the economy. Energy efficiency also lowers operating expenses, allowing providers to invest more in high-quality, affordable health care.

Mitigating the impacts of climate change is a collective effort. That's why Kaiser Permanente is part of a coalition of health-care organizations, led by Health Care Without Harm, that advocates for broad solutions to climate change.

It's time for the public health community—and, indeed, all parts of our society—to rise to this challenge. Lives depend on our response to climate change. Without a healthy planet, we can't hope to have healthy people living on it.

Conclusion

ADOPTING A PRECISION APPROACH TO COMMUNITY HEALTH holds enormous promise. By taking advantage of new technologies and methods, we can improve the lives of everyone in this country. I had a chance to witness the impact this approach made in Chicago. I saw the needle moving in the right direction on a number of significant health challenges, and that progress is now continuing in many other places as well.

Public health champions such as Oxiris Barbot in New York, Barbara Ferrer in Los Angeles County, and Julie Morita in Chicago are doing amazing work, employing data, media, policy, and community-level interventions to serve all, but especially the most vulnerable and disenfranchised. As the health commissioner of New York City, Dr. Barbot has been leading a transformational agenda, including prioritizing mental health and implementing progressive tobacco policies. As I did, Dr. Barbot saw how lack of economic opportunity and poor housing damages health while she was working as a clinician. She treated patients with severe asthma who were using their stoves for heat and hoped a doctor's note would help them move higher on the list for housing assistance. "That's not a way to treat a chronic health condition," she said.

Dr. Ferrer, who directs the four-thousand-person public health department in Los Angeles County, has also made equity a top priority, citing higher infant mortality rates and shorter life spans for black residents as one of the region's biggest challenges. Her department is working to improve health outcomes with a broad range of tools, including targeted community-level interventions. I have been particularly impressed with their focus on sexually transmitted infections.

My successor in Chicago, Dr. Morita, took the precision community health approach to the next level with Healthy Chicago 2.0. Step one is identifying the most vulnerable communities, understanding the challenges they face, and delivering appropriate care in a timely fashion. Step two is ensuring that our social and physical environments support rather than threaten health. Even though Julie has transitioned to the Robert Wood Johnson Foundation to lead its nationwide programming, the work in Chicago is continuing under the leadership of Mayor Lori Lightfoot.

The fundamental strength of precision community health is that it can address the key question of health equity: Are we creating the right environment so that people who are the most vulnerable can have the best chances for healthy and productive lives?

To ensure that the answer is yes, we have to take advantage of the new industrial revolution that is currently blurring the lines between the physical, digital, and biological spheres. We can leverage nanotechnology, the Internet of Things, artificial intelligence, and other radical advances to improve community health around the world.

The new industrial revolution is happening whether we like it or not. Less certain is the revolution in public health, with a goal of promoting health and health equity rather than just preventing disease. For it to be truly transformative, we need a social movement that changes our understanding of health. As we have seen, public health is much more than simply a broadened version of clinical medicine. We will need to come to grips with the direct and indirect effects that social, fiscal, and environmental policies; our approach to education; and the state of our housing and other infrastructure all have on our health. A new kind of civic activism, which is already beginning to appear in some places, will be necessary to fulfill the promise of precision community health.

New Challenges Await

Precision community health, no matter how powerful an idea it may be in the abstract, will do little to affect the lives of real people without all of us in some way rethinking our assumptions about how technology and community intersect in the twenty-first century. Practitioners of precision community health, like all public health officials since the nineteenth century, will need to address unexpected and urgent problems, be they changes in behavior or natural disasters, and they will need to bring new tools to the job. But they will also need to apply those tools to solving broader systemic problems that are unique to our time, such as privacy versus open data, and climate change.

This precision approach to community health offers new insights into age-old problems such as hurricanes and wildfires. Now we have a deeper appreciation of how such natural disasters can shape the lives of those with the fewest resources: the young, the elderly, and those living in poverty. Hurricane Katrina and then Hurricane Maria in Puerto Rico made us all painfully aware of the fact that inequalities make people more vulnerable and revealed how much work we still have to do.

The California wildfires, such as the Camp Fire, the deadliest and most destructive wildfire in California history, which destroyed the town of Paradise in the fall of 2018, put the profound impacts of such disasters on public health into even starker relief. The fires and mudslides that followed left thousands homeless, and many residents will not be able to rebuild. Health is not possible if people don't have a safe place to call home.

Other challenges are more diffuse but no less urgent.

Back in 2012, I became increasingly concerned about e-cigarettes. Most people at that time didn't even know what these devices were. In Chicago, we started a campaign to educate the public about them. The public health community hadn't yet agreed on a clear position, especially given that many scholars thought e-cigarettes could be less deadly than their combustible counterparts. Why not adopt a risk reduction approach and help smokers give up combustible cigarettes? I wasn't opposed to that philosophy. What concerned me, however, was the fact that e-cigarettes, with their kids-enticing flavors, were being used to lure children and create another generation of nicotine-addicted people.

I knew that Big Tobacco would end up the main player in the e-cigarette business. But when we introduced the e-cigarette regulation in 2013, little did we know that Juul products would be so popular among high school students. Little did we know that people would be hospitalized and many would die from vaping-related pneumonia. In August 2019, the chief executive officer of Juul Labs stepped down and was replaced by a senior executive of Altria, one of the world's largest producers of cigarettes and parent company of Phillip Morris USA.

Today, vaping is a major public health issue, and local governments across the country and many states have introduced new regulations to build on what we introduced back in Chicago in 2013. The federal government, including the Food and Drug Administration (FDA), is weighing in. Mayor Rahm Emanuel and I called on the FDA in 2013 and 2014 to act and regulate e-cigarettes. Little was done then. Now even Congress is hosting a series of hearings to better understand the role it can play in confronting this public health threat.

Each of these challenges, and those we have yet to anticipate, will require government engagement and a willingness by public health officials to use new tools and try new approaches. Big cities such as New York, Los Angeles, and Chicago will continue to be centers for innovative solutions, and now is the time to invest in their efforts. We must think and act systemically if we want to create real change. No single measure will suffice to solve complex health problems, whether they are novel or long-standing.

The Path Forward

Supporting local health departments will be critical to advancing a precision community health approach across the country. So will funding effective state health departments and an adaptive Centers for Disease Control and Prevention (CDC). This is about making an investment in our public agencies, allocating the resources needed to support innovative public health efforts. It's about training staff to equip our workforce with the new skills they will need to advance the field. It's also about enhancing our data systems across the country.

Our public health departments and, indeed, public health as a profession must evolve to broaden its focus from medical treatment to wellness. But just as individual health happens outside the doctor's office, public health happens outside agency walls. A social movement to think broadly about health is a must at this point. Health is not just about individual behavior. It's about how we behave as a community. It's about the policies we put in place. It's about the systems we create. It's about the environments we engineer. Precision community health is all about reshaping these policies, systems, and environments so that everyone in this world has an opportunity to thrive.

But even that is not enough.

There are still billions of people in world, including tens of millions of people here in the United States, who are struggling daily to meet their basic human needs. In a nationally representative survey commissioned by Kaiser Permanente in 2019, 68 percent of people living in this country had to face at least one unmet social need in the prior year. For 25 percent of people, that social need was a barrier to health. Think about it. That's 25 percent of people in this country who had to make a choice between buying milk and getting their medications. They had to choose between paying their rent and paying their medical bill.

Precision community health offers the best promise to address these issues upstream, while delivering immediate care to vulnerable populations. Unmet social needs have a direct impact on health. You can't eat well if you can't afford nutritious groceries. You can't get appropriate medical care if you don't have transportation to your doctor's office. If you don't have access to safe streets or parks, exercise becomes a lot more difficult. If you are struggling with social isolation, you won't be able to thrive. That's why addressing individuals' social health is critical to addressing their physical health and mental health. It is time to understand health as a societal endeavor rather than simply a personal one.

People are only as healthy as their community. Precision community health can improve the well-being of both. It is an opportunity we cannot fail to grasp.

Acknowledgments

I would like to acknowledge my colleagues from the Chicago Department of Public Health for embracing the evolution of public health and the people of Kaiser Permanente for taking community health to the next level. And a big thank-you to Jonathan Adams, whose support was critical to getting this book published.

Notes

Introduction

1. Muin J. Khoury, Michael F. Iademarco, and William T. Riley, "Precision Public Health for the Era of Precision Medicine," *American Journal of Preventive Medicine* 50, no. 3 (2016): 398–401, https://doi.org/10.1016/j.amepre.2015.08.031; Merlin Chowkwanyun, Ronald Bayer, and Sandro Galea, "'Precision' Public Health—between Novelty and Hype," *New England Journal of Medicine* 379, no. 15 (October 11, 2018): 1398–1400, https://doi.org/10.1056/NEJMp1806634.

Chapter 1. Public Health in Chicago and Beyond

1. Raj Chetty et al., "The Opportunity Atlas: Mapping the Childhood Roots of Social Mobility," October 2018, https://opportunityinsights.org/wp-content/uploads/2018/10/atlas_paper.pdf.
2. Chicago Department of Public Health, "Healthy Chicago: A Public Health Agenda for a Healthy City, Healthy Neighborhoods, Healthy People, and Healthy Homes," December 29, 2010, https://www.chicago.gov/dam/city/depts/cdph/CDPH/PublicHlthAgenda2011.pdf.
3. University of Wisconsin Population Health Institute, "2019 County Health Rankings Key Findings Report," 2019, https://www.countyhealthrankings.org/reports/2019-county-health-rankings-key-findings-report.
4. John Duffy, *The Sanitarians: A History of American Public Health* (Urbana: University of Illinois Press, 1990).
5. John Duffy, *Epidemics in Colonial America* (Port Washington, NY: Kennikat Press, 1972).
6. John Duffy, *A History of Public Health in New York City, 1625–1866*, vol. 1 (New York: Russell Sage Foundation, 1968), https://muse.jhu.edu/books/9781610441643/.

7. Duffy, *Sanitarians*.

8. Meyer Friedman and Gerald W. Friedland, *Medicine's 10 Greatest Discoveries* (New Haven, CT: Yale University Press, 2000).

9. Stefan Riedel, "Edward Jenner and the History of Smallpox and Vaccination," *Baylor University Medical Center Proceedings* 18, no. 1 (January 2005): 21–25, https://doi.org/10.1080/08998280.2005.11928028.

10. Richard B. Fisher, *Edward Jenner, 1749–1823* (and Per-Olof Östergren, 1991).

11. Robin A. Weiss and José Esparza, "The Prevention and Eradication of Smallpox: A Commentary on Sloane (1755) 'An Account of Inoculation.'" *Philosophical Transactions of the Royal Society B: Biological Sciences* 370, no. 1666 (April 19, 2015), https://doi.org/10.1098/rstb.2014.0378.

12. Duffy, *Sanitarians*.

13. Russell Frank Weigley, Nicholas B. Wainwright, and Edwin Wolf, *Philadelphia: A 300-Year History* (New York: Norton, 1982).

14. Dirk J. Struik, *The Origins of American Science* (New York: Cameron, 1957).

15. Lemuel Shattuck, *Report of the Sanitary Commission of Massachusetts, 1850* (Cambridge, MA: Harvard University Press, 1948).

16. C.-E. A. Winslow, "The Message of Lemuel Shattuck for 1948," *American Journal of Public Health* 39, no. 2 (February 1, 1949): 156–62, https://doi.org/10.2105/AJPH.39.2.156.

17. Duffy, *Sanitarians*.

18. Charles E. Rosenberg, *The Cholera Years: The United States in 1832, 1849, and 1866* (Chicago: University of Chicago Press, 1962).

19. Thomas Neville Bonner, *Medicine in Chicago, 1850–1950: A Chapter in the Social and Scientific Development of a City* (Urbana: University of Illinois Press, 1991), https://catalog.hathitrust.org/Record/002476917.

20. Libby Hill, *The Chicago River: A Natural and Unnatural History* (Chicago: Lake Claremont Press, 2000).

21. Ron Grossman, "Raising Chicago out of the Mud," *Chicago Tribune*, November 9, 2015, https://www.chicagotribune.com/news/history/ct-raising-chicago-streets-flashback-1122-jm-20151118-story.html; https://www.chicagomag.com/Chicago-Magazine/August-2010/Raising-Chicago-An-Illustrated-History/.

22. Louis P. Cain, "The Search for an Optimum Sanitation Jurisdiction: The Metropolitan Sanitary District of Greater Chicago; A Case Study," Essays

in Public Works History series, no. 10 (Washington, DC: Public Works Historical Society, 1980).

23. Robert Cromie, *The Great Chicago Fire* (New York: McGraw-Hill, 1958).

24. Donald L. Miller, *City of the Century: The Epic of Chicago and the Making of America* (New York: Simon & Schuster, 1996).

25. Jennifer Koslow, "Public Health," *Encyclopedia of Chicago*, 2004, http://www.encyclopedia.chicagohistory.org/pages/1020.html.

26. Bonner, *Medicine in Chicago*.

27. Quoted in Bonner, *Medicine in Chicago*, 22.

28. Margaret Garb, "Health, Morality, and Housing: The 'Tenement Problem' in Chicago," *American Journal of Public Health* 93, no. 9 (September 10, 2003): 1420–30, https://doi.org/10.2105/AJPH.93.9.1420.

29. Hill, *Chicago River*.

Chapter 2. Learning the Hard Way

1. Robert J. Sampson, *Great American City: Chicago and the Enduring Neighborhood Effect* (Chicago: University of Chicago Press, 2012).

2. Edward Glaeser and Jacob Vigdor, "The End of the Segregated Century: Racial Separation in America's Neighborhoods, 1890–2010," Civic Report 66 (New York: Center for State and Local Leadership, Manhattan Institute for Policy Research, 2012), https://media4.manhattan-institute.org/pdf/cr_66.pdf.

3. S. V. Subramanian, Tony Blakely, and Ichiro Kawachi, "Income Inequality as a Public Health Concern: Where Do We Stand? Commentary on 'Is Exposure to Income Inequality a Public Health Concern?,'" pt. 1, *Health Services Research* 38, no. 1 (February 2003): 153–67, https://doi.org/10.1111/1475-6773.00110.

4. Organisation for Economic Co-operation and Development, "Crisis Squeezes Income and Puts Pressure on Inequality and Poverty" (Paris: OECD, 2013), http://www.oecd.org/els/soc/OECD2013-Inequality-and-Poverty-8p.pdf.

5. National Academies of Sciences, Engineering, and Medicine, *The Growing Gap in Life Expectancy by Income: Implications for Federal Programs and Policy Responses* (Washington, DC: National Academies Press, 2015), https://doi.org/10.17226/19015.

6. Samuel L. Dickman, David U. Himmelstein, and Steffie Woolhandler, "Inequality and the Health-Care System in the USA," *Lancet* 389, no. 10077 (April 8, 2017): 1431–41, https://doi.org/10.1016/S0140-6736(17)30398-7.

7. National Academies of Sciences, Engineering, and Medicine, *Communities in Action: Pathways to Health Equity* (Washington, DC: National Academies Press, 2017), https://doi.org/10.17226/24624.

8. Zinzi D. Bailey et al., "Structural Racism and Health Inequities in the USA: Evidence and Interventions," *Lancet* 389, no. 10077 (April 8, 2017): 1453–63, https://doi.org/10.1016/S0140-6736(17)30569-X.

9. US Environmental Protection Agency, Office of Inspector General, "Management Weaknesses Delayed Response to Flint Water Crisis," report no. 18-P-0221, July 19, 2018, accessed April 11, 2019, https://www.epa.gov/office-inspector-general/report-management-weaknesses-delayed-response-flint-water-crisis.

10. Mona Hanna-Attisha et al., "Elevated Blood Lead Levels in Children Associated with the Flint Drinking Water Crisis: A Spatial Analysis of Risk and Public Health Response," *American Journal of Public Health* 106, no. 2 (February 1, 2016): 283–90, https://doi.org/10.2105/AJPH.2015.303003.

11. Michelle L. Bell and Keita Ebisu, "Environmental Inequality in Exposures to Airborne Particulate Matter Components in the United States," *Environmental Health Perspectives* 120, no. 12 (December 1, 2012): 1699–1704, https://doi.org/10.1289/ehp.1205201.

12. Thomas A. LaVeist, Darrell Gaskin, and Patrick Richard, "Estimating the Economic Burden of Racial Health Inequalities in the United States," *International Journal of Health Services* 41, no. 2 (April 1, 2011): 231–38, accessed September 21, 2018, https://doi.org/10.2190/HS.41.2.c.

13. Timothy A. Waidmann, "Estimating the Cost of Racial and Ethnic Health Disparities" (Washington, DC: Urban Institute, September 2009), https://www.urban.org/research/publication/estimating-cost-racial-and-ethnic-health-disparities.

14. Steven H. Woolf et al., "How Are Income and Wealth Linked to Health and Longevity?" (Washington, DC: Urban Institute, April 13, 2015), https://www.urban.org/research/publication/how-are-income-and-wealth-linked-health-and-longevity.

15. Philip P. Goodney et al., "Variation in the Care of Surgical Conditions: Diabetes and Peripheral Arterial Disease," report of the Dartmouth Atlas Project (Hanover, NH: Dartmouth Institute for Health Policy and Clinical Practice, 2014), http://www.dartmouthatlas.org/downloads/reports/Diabetes_report_10_14_14.pdf.

16. Amy L. Fairchild and Ava Alkon, "Back to the Future? Diabetes, HIV, and the Boundaries of Public Health," *Journal of Health Politics, Policy and Law* 32, no. 4 (August 1, 2007): 561–93, https://doi.org/10.1215/03616878-2007-017.

17. Ross C. Brownson, Jonathan E. Fielding, and Christopher M. Maylahn, "Evidence-Based Public Health: A Fundamental Concept for Public Health Practice," *Annual Review of Public Health* 30, no. 1 (April 21, 2009): 175–201, https://doi.org/10.1146/annurev.publhealth.031308.100134.

18. Emily Laflamme et al., "Life Expectancy in Chicago, 1990–2010," Healthy Chicago Reports (Chicago: Chicago Department of Public Health, June 2014), https://www.cityofchicago.org/content/dam/city/depts/cdph/statistics_and_reports/LifeExpectancyinChicago1990-2010.pdf.

19. Kinsey Hasstedt, "Federally Qualified Health Centers: Vital Sources of Care, No Substitute for the Family Planning Safety Net," *Guttmacher Policy Review* 20 (2017), https://www.guttmacher.org/gpr/2017/05/federally-qualified-health-centers-vital-sources-care-no-substitute-family-planning.

20. Vincent J. Felitti et al., "Relationship of Childhood Abuse and Household Dysfunction to Many of the Leading Causes of Death in Adults," *American Journal of Preventive Medicine* 14, no. 4 (May 1, 1998): 245–58, https://doi.org/10.1016/S0749-3797(98)00017-8.

21. National Association of County and City Health Officials, "2013 National Profile of Local Health Departments" (Washington, DC: NACCHO, January 2014), http://nacchoprofilestudy.org/wp-content/uploads/2014/02/2013_National_Profile021014.pdf.

22. Gary Slutkin, "Violence Is a Contagious Disease," in Institute of Medicine and National Research Council, *Contagion of Violence: Workshop Summary* (Washington, DC: National Academies Press, 2013), 94–111, https://www.ncbi.nlm.nih.gov/books/NBK207245/.

23. Slutkin, "Violence Is a Contagious Disease."

Chapter 3. Building Coalitions

1. Paula Braveman and Laura Gottlieb, "The Social Determinants of Health: It's Time to Consider the Causes of the Causes," *Public Health Reports* 129, no. 1, suppl. 2 (2014): 19–31, https://doi.org/10.1177/00333549141291S206.

2. Penelope Hawe and Alan Shiell, "Social Capital and Health Promotion: A Review," *Social Science & Medicine* 51, no. 6 (September 15, 2000): 871–85, https://doi.org/10.1016/S0277-9536(00)00067-8.

3. Centers for Disease Control and Prevention, "Community Profile: Chicago, Illinois," https://www.cdc.gov/nccdphp/dch/programs/communities puttingpreventiontowork/communities/profiles/both-il_chicago .htm; Chicago Department of Public Health, "Overweight and Obesity among Chicago Public Schools Students, 2010–11," https://www .chicago.gov/content/dam/city/depts/cdph/CDPH/OverweightObesity ReportFeb272013.pdf.

4. Glen P. Mays, Cezar B. Mamaril, and Lava R. Timsina, "Preventable Death Rates Fell Where Communities Expanded Population Health Activities through Multisector Networks," *Health Affairs* 35, no. 11 (November 2, 2016): 2005–13, https://doi.org/10.1377/hlthaff.2016.0848.

5. National Academies of Sciences, Engineering, and Medicine, *Communities in Action: Pathways to Health Equity* (Washington, DC: National Academies Press, 2017), https://doi.org/10.17226/24624.

6. Katherine M. Keyes and Sandro Galea, *Population Health Science* (New York: Oxford University Press, 2016).

7. Richard A. Goodman, Rebecca Bunnell, and Samuel F. Posner, "What Is 'Community Health'? Examining the Meaning of an Evolving Field in Public Health," *Preventive Medicine* 67, suppl. 1 (October 2014): S58–S61, https://doi.org/10.1016/j.ypmed.2014.07.028.

8. Public Health Accreditation Board, Standards and Measures, version 1.5, December 2013, https://www.phaboard.org/wp-content/uploads/2019/01/PHABSM_WEB_LR1.pdf.

9. Robert D. Putnam, *Bowling Alone: The Collapse and Revival of American Community* (New York: Simon & Schuster, 2000).

10. John G. Bruhn and Stewart Wolf, *The Roseto Story: An Anatomy of Health* (Norman: University of Oklahoma Press, 1979).

11. Émile Durkheim, *Suicide: A Study in Sociology*, trans. John A. Spaulding and George Simpson (Glencoe, IL: Free Press, 1951).

12. James A. Wiley and Terry C. Camacho, "Life-style and Future Health: Evidence from the Alameda County Study," *Preventive Medicine* 9, no. 1 (January 1980): 1–21, https://doi.org/10.1016/0091-7435(80)90056-0.

13. Lisa F. Berkman and S. Leonard Syme, "Social Networks, Host Resistance, and Mortality: A Nine-Year Follow-Up Study of Alameda County Residents," *American Journal of Epidemiology* 109, no. 2 (February 1979): 186–204, https://doi.org/10.1093/oxfordjournals.aje.a112674.

14. Francis Fukuyama, "Social Capital and Civil Society," IMF Working Paper WP/00/74 (Washington, DC: International Monetary Fund, 2000), https://www.imf.org/en/Publications/WP/Issues/2016/12/30/Social -Capital-and-Civil-Society-3547.

15. S. E. D. Shortt, "Making Sense of Social Capital, Health, and Policy," *Health Policy* 70, no. 1 (October 2004): 11–22, https://doi.org/10.1016/ j.healthpol.2004.01.007.

16. Ichiro Kawachi, Bruce P. Kennedy, and Richard G. Wilkinson, "Crime: Social Disorganization and Relative Deprivation," *Social Science & Medicine* 48, no. 6 (March 1, 1999): 719–31, https://doi.org/10.1016/S0277 -9536(98)00400-6; Martin Lindström, Bertil S. Hanson, and Per-Olof Östergren, "Socioeconomic Differences in Leisure-Time Physical Activity: The Role of Social Participation and Social Capital in Shaping Health Related Behaviour," *Social Science & Medicine* 52, no. 3 (February 2001): 441–51, https://doi.org/10.1016/S0277-9536(00)00153-2.

17. Michael S. Hendryx et al., "Access to Health Care and Community Social Capital," *Health Services Research* 37, no. 1 (February 2002): 85–101, https://doi.org/10.1111/1475-6773.00111.

18. R. Rosenheck et al., "Service Delivery and Community: Social Capital, Service Systems Integration, and Outcomes among Homeless Persons with Severe Mental Illness," *Health Services Research* 36, no. 4 (August 2001): 691–710, http://www.ncbi.nlm.nih.gov/pubmed/11508635.

19. I. Kawachi et al., "Social Capital, Income Inequality, and Mortality," *American Journal of Public Health* 87, no. 9 (September 1, 1997): 1491–98, https://ajph.aphapublications.org/doi/abs/10.2105/AJPH.87.9.1491.

20. Mays, Mamaril, and Timsina, "Preventable Death Rates," 2007.

21. Danaei Goodarz et al., "The Promise of Prevention: The Effects of Four Preventable Risk Factors on National Life Expectancy and Life Expectancy Disparities by Race and County in the United States," *PLoS Medicine*

7, no. 3 (March 23, 2010): e1000248, https://doi.org/10.1371/journal
.pmed.1000248.

22. Goodman, Bunnell, and Posner, "What Is 'Community Health'?"

23. M. P. Stern et al., "Results of a Two-Year Health Education Campaign on
Dietary Behavior: The Stanford Three Community Study," *Circulation*
54, no. 5 (November 1, 1976): 826–33, https://doi.org/10.1161/01.CIR
.54.5.826; Stephen P. Fortmann et al., "Community Intervention Trials:
Reflections on the Stanford Five-City Project Experience," *American Journal of Epidemiology* 142, no. 6 (September 15, 1995): 576–86, https://doi
.org/10.1093/oxfordjournals.aje.a117678.

24. Fortmann et al., "Community Intervention Trials."

25. Marshall W. Kreuter, "PATCH: Its Origin, Basic Concepts, and Links to
Contemporary Public Health Policy," *Journal of Health Education* 23, no. 3
(1992): 135–39, https://doi.org/10.1080/10556699.1992.10616276.

26. Robin E. Soler, Kathleen L. Whitten, and Phyllis G. Ottley, "Communities Putting Prevention to Work: Local Evaluation of Community-Based
Strategies Designed to Make Healthy Living Easier," *Preventive Medicine* 67, suppl. 1 (October 1, 2014): S1–S3, https://doi.org/10.1016/J
.YPMED.2014.08.020.

27. Metropolitan Chicago Breast Cancer Task Force, "Improving Quality and
Reducing Disparities in Breast Cancer Mortality in Metropolitan Chicago," October 2007, http://www.chicagobreastcancer.org/site/files/904/
100490/352501/748152/Task_Force_Report,_October_2007.pdf.

28. Dominique Sighoko et al., "Changes in the Racial Disparity in Breast
Cancer Mortality in the Ten US Cities with the Largest African American
Populations from 1999 to 2013: The Reduction in Breast Cancer Mortality Disparity in Chicago," *Cancer Causes & Control* 28, no. 6 (June 2017):
563–68, https://doi.org/10.1007/s10552-017-0878-y.

29. City of Chicago, Department of Housing and Economic Development,
"A Recipe for Healthy Places: Addressing the Intersection of Food and
Obesity in Chicago," 2013, https://www.chicago.gov/city/en/depts/dcd/
supp_info/a_recipe_for_healthyplaces.html.

30. Mays, Mamaril, and Timsina, "Preventable Death Rates."

31. Mays, Mamaril, and Timsina, "Preventable Death Rates."

Chapter 4. Tapping the Power of Big Data

1. Ithiel de Sola Pool, "Tracking the Flow of Information," *Science* 221, no. 4611 (August 12, 1983): 609–13, https://doi.org/10.1126/science .221.4611.609.

2. John Duffy, *The Sanitarians: A History of American Public Health* (Urbana: University of Illinois Press, 1992).

3. Lester Breslow, "Multiphasic Screening Examinations: An Extension of the Mass Screening Technique," *American Journal of Public Health* 40 (March 1950): 274–78, https://www.ncbi.nlm.nih.gov/pmc/articles/ PMC1528443/pdf/amjphnation01018-0027.pdf.

4. Morris F. Collen, "Periodic Health Examinations Using an Automated Multitest Laboratory," *JAMA* 195, no. 10 (March 7, 1966): 830, https:// doi.org/10.1001/jama.1966.03100100082023.

5. Marion Ball, Donald Lindberg, and Izet Masic, "Special Tribute on Morris F. Collen: Charismatic Leader of Medical Informatics," *Acta Informatica Medica* 22, no. 1 (February 2014): 4–5, https://doi.org/10.5455/aim.2014.22.4-5.

6. Andrew Friede, Henrik L. Blum, and Mike McDonald, "Public Health Informatics: How Information-Age Technology Can Strengthen Public Health," *Annual Review of Public Health* 16, no. 1 (May 1995): 239–52, https://doi.org/10.1146/annurev.pu.16.050195.001323.

7. Leslie Lenert and David N. Sundwall, "Public Health Surveillance and Meaningful Use Regulations: A Crisis of Opportunity," *American Journal of Public Health* 102, no. 3 (March 1, 2012): e1–e7, https://doi.org/10 .2105/AJPH.2011.300542.

8. Merlin Chowkwanyun, Ronald Bayer, and Sandro Galea, "'Precision' Public Health—between Novelty and Hype," *New England Journal of Medicine* 379, no. 15 (October 11, 2018): 1398–1400, http://dx.doi.org/10 .1056/NEJMp1806634.

9. Scott F. Dowell, David Blazes, and Susan Desmond-Hellmann, "Four Steps to Precision Public Health," *Nature* 540, no. 7632 (December 5, 2016): 189–91, https://doi.org/10.1038/540189a.

10. Elaine Grant, "The Promise of Big Data," *Harvard Public Health* (Spring/ Summer 2012), https://www.hsph.harvard.edu/news/magazine/spr12-big -data-tb-health-costs/.

11. Marshall Allen, "Health Insurers Are Vacuuming Up Details about You—and It Could Raise Your Rates," *Shots: Health News from NPR*,

July 17, 2018, https://www.npr.org/sections/health-shots/2018/07/17/629441555/health-insurers-are-vacuuming-up-details-about-you-and-it-could-raise-your-rates.

12. National Academies of Sciences, Engineering, and Medicine, *To Err Is Human: Building a Safer Health System* (Washington, DC: National Academies Press, 2000), https://doi.org/10.17226/9728.

13. D. L. Sackett et al., "Evidence Based Medicine: What It Is and What It Isn't," *BMJ* 312, no. 7023 (January 13, 1996): 71–72, https://doi.org/10.1136/bmj.312.7023.71.

14. Hamilton Moses et al., "Financial Anatomy of Biomedical Research," *JAMA* 294, no. 11 (September 21, 2005): 1333–42, https://doi.org/10.1001/jama.294.11.1333.

15. LeighAnne Olsen, Dara Aisner, and J. Michael McGinnis, eds., *The Learning Healthcare System: Workshop Summary* (Washington, DC: National Academies Press, 2007), 3.

16. Jennifer A. Bernstein et al., "Ensuring Public Health's Future in a National-Scale Learning Health System," *American Journal of Preventive Medicine* 48, no. 4 (April 2015): 480–87, https://doi.org/10.1016/j.amepre.2014.11.013.

17. Kaiser Permanente, "Historic Kaiser Permanente Data to Aid in Long-Term Study to Determine Extent of Ethnic Disparities in Brain Health and Dementia," news release, July 13, 2016, https://www.prnewswire.com/news-releases/historic-kaiser-permanente-data-to-aid-in-long-term-study-to-determine-extent-of-ethnic-disparities-in-brain-health-and-dementia-300297820.html.

18. Jenine K. Harris et al., "Health Department Use of Social Media to Identify Foodborne Illness—Chicago, Illinois, 2013–2014," *Centers for Disease Control and Prevention Morbidity and Mortality Weekly Report* 63, no. 32 (August 15, 2014): 681–85, https://www.cdc.gov/mmwr/pdf/wk/mm6332.pdf.

19. Sean Thornton, "A Profile of Technology and Innovation in Chicago," Harvard Kennedy School Ash Center for Democratic Governance and Innovation, Data-Smart City Solutions, April 11, 2013, https://datasmart.ash.harvard.edu/news/article/a-profile-of-technology-and-innovation-in-chicago-190.

20. Michael Hawthorne, "Lead Paint Poisons Poor Chicago Kids as City Spends Millions Less on Cleanup," *Chicago Tribune*, May 1, 2015, https://

www.chicagotribune.com/investigations/ct-lead-poisoning-chicago-met
-20150501-story.html.

21. Eric Potash et al., "Predictive Modeling for Public Health: Preventing Childhood Lead Poisoning," in *Proceedings of the 21st ACM SIGKDD International Conference on Knowledge Discovery and Data Mining*, 2039–47 (New York: Association for Computing Machinery, 2015), accessed November 5, 2018, https://doi.org/10.1145/2783258 .2788629.

22. J. Brew et al., "Chicago Department of Public Health: Data-Driven Strategies for Lead Poisoning Prevention," paper presented at the Eric and Wendy Schultz Data Science for Social Good Symposium, Chicago, 2014.

23. Computation Institute, "Data Science for Social Good 2014—Chapter 2," YouTube video, 3:25, https://www.youtube.com/watch?v=Fc4IHhJSV3I &feature=youtu.be.

Chapter 5. Rise above the Noise

1. Jenine K. Harris et al., "Tweeting for and against Public Health Policy: Response to the Chicago Department of Public Health's Electronic Cigarette Twitter Campaign," *Journal of Medical Internet Research* 16, no. 10 (October 2014): e238, https://doi.org/10.2196/jmir.3622.

2. Kim Bellware, "Chicago E-Cigarette Ban Could Get Snuffed Out by Surprising City Council Pushback to Rahm's Plan," *Huffington Post*, December 13, 2013.

3. Peter Hajek et al., "A Randomized Trial of E-Cigarettes versus Nicotine-Replacement Therapy," *New England Journal of Medicine* 380, no. 7 (February 14, 2019): 629–37, https://doi.org/10.1056/NEJMoa1808779.

4. American Nonsmokers' Rights Foundation, "States and Municipalities with Laws Regulating Use of Electronic Cigarettes as of July 1, 2019," http://no-smoke.org/wp-content/uploads/pdf/ecigslaws.pdf.

5. California Department of Public Health, Still Blowing Smoke, https:// stillblowingsmoke.org/.

6. NOT Blowing Smoke, http://notblowingsmoke.org.

7. Sheila Kaplan and Matt Richtel, "Juul Closes Deal with Tobacco Giant Altria," *New York Times*, December 20, 2018, https://www.nytimes.com/ 2018/12/20/health/juul-reaches-deal-with-tobacco-giant-altria.html.

8. Martin McKee et al., "The Debate on Electronic Cigarettes," *Lancet* 384, no. 9960 (December 13, 2014): 2107, https://doi.org/10.1016/S0140 -6736(14)62366-7.

9. Jenine K. Harris et al., "Health Department Use of Social Media to Identify Foodborne Illness—Chicago, Illinois, 2013–2014," *Centers for Disease Control and Prevention Morbidity and Mortality Weekly Report* 63, no. 32 (August 15, 2014): 681–85, https://www.cdc.gov/mmwr/pdf/wk/ mm6332.pdf.

10. G. A. Giovino et al., "Differential Trends in Cigarette Smoking in the USA: Is Menthol Slowing Progress?," *Tobacco Control* 24, no. 1 (January 2015): 28–37, http://dx.doi.org/10.1136/tobaccocontrol-2013-051159.

11. Substance Abuse and Mental Health Services Administration, Office of Applied Studies, "The NSDUH Report: Recent Trends in Menthol Cigarette Use" (Rockville, MD: SAMHSA, 2009), https://www.samhsa.gov/ data/report/nsduh-report-recent-trends-menthol-cigarette-use.

12. Substance Abuse and Mental Health Services Administration, "NSDUH Report," fig. 1.

13. US Department of Health and Human Services, *Preventing Tobacco Use among Youth and Young Adults: A Report of the Surgeon General* (Atlanta, GA: USDHHS, Centers for Disease Control and Prevention, National Center for Chronic Disease Prevention and Health Promotion, Office on Smoking and Health, 2012), https://www.ncbi.nlm.nih.gov/books/ NBK99237/.

14. Rod McCullom, "Can Chicago Curb Menthol Smoking among African-American Youth?," *Scientific American*, March 19, 2014, https://www .scientificamerican.com/article/can-chicago-curb-menthol-smoking -among-african-american-youth/.

15. Dave Tabler, "Light Up a Spud!," *Appalachian History: Stories, Quotes, and Anecdotes* (blog), July 19, 2018, http://www.appalachianhistory.net/2018/ 07/light-up-spud.html.

16. Phillip S. Gardiner, "The African Americanization of Menthol Cigarette Use in the United States," *Nicotine & Tobacco Research* 6, suppl. 1 (February 2004): S55–S65, https://doi.org/10.1080/14622200310001649478.

17. Kathleen R. Stratton et al., eds., *Clearing the Smoke: Assessing the Science Base for Tobacco Harm Reduction* (Washington, DC: National Academy Press, 2001).

18. Gardiner, "African Americanization of Menthol Cigarette Use."

19. Richard W. Pollay, Jung S. Lee, and David Carter-Whitney, "Separate, but Not Equal: Racial Segmentation in Cigarette Advertising," *Journal of Advertising* 21, no. 1 (March 1, 1992): 45–57, https://doi.org/10.1080/00913367.1992.10673359.

20. Quoted in Phillip Gardiner and Pamela Clark, "Summary of the Second Conference on Menthol Cigarettes: *Menthol in Cigarettes: It Helps the Poison Go Down Easier*, A Report to the Food and Drug Administration (FDA) Prepared as Public Comment," December 21, 2009, 23, https://cdn.ymaws.com/www.naquitline.org/resource/resmgr/news/100202_menthol-cigarette-rep.pdf.

21. Jonathan P. Winickoff et al., "US Attitudes about Banning Menthol in Cigarettes: Results from a Nationally Representative Survey," *American Journal of Public Health* 101, no. 7 (July 1, 2011): 1234–36, https://doi.org/10.2105/AJPH.2011.300146.

22. Joseph G. L. Lee et al., "Promotion of Tobacco Use Cessation for Lesbian, Gay, Bisexual, and Transgender People: A Systematic Review," *American Journal of Preventive Medicine* 47, no. 6 (December 2014): 823–31, https://doi.org/10.1016/j.amepre.2014.07.051.

23. Phoenix Alicia Matthews et al., "SBM Recommends Policy Support to Reduce Smoking Disparities for Sexual and Gender Minorities," *Translational Behavioral Medicine* 8, no. 5 (October 2018): 692–95, https://doi.org/10.1093/tbm/ibx017.

24. Lee et al., "Promotion of Tobacco Use Cessation."

25. Illinois Department of Public Health, Division of Vital Records, "Chicago Teen Birth Rate, 2010–2015," https://www.healthychicagobabies.org/wp-content/uploads/2017/11/Teen-Birth-Rate-edited2015_final.pdf.

26. Philip Kleinman, *Saatchi & Saatchi: The Inside Story* (Lincolnwood, IL: NTC Business Books, 1989).

27. The Bridgespan Group, "Needle-Moving Community Collaboratives: Case Study: Milwaukee," February 6, 2012, https://www.bridgespan.org/bridgespan/Images/articles/needle-moving-community-collaboratives/profiles/community-collaboratives-case-study-milwaukee.pdf.

28. Kyla Calvert Mason, "Milwaukee's Teen Birth Rate Drops to Historic Low," Wisconsin Public Radio, October 28, 2016, https://www.wpr.org/milwaukees-teen-birth-rate-drops-historic-low.

29. Kate Dries, "Chicago Is the Latest City to Tackle Teen Pregnancy with Weird Ads," *Jezebel*, May 20, 2013, https://jezebel.com/chicago-is-the -latest-city-to-tackle-teen-pregnancy-wit-508902075.

Chapter 6. Challenge the Status Quo

1. Karen A. Cullen et al., "Notes from the Field: Use of Electronic Cigarettes and Any Tobacco Product among Middle and High School Students—United States, 2011–2018," *Centers for Disease Control and Prevention Morbidity and Mortality Weekly Report* 67, no. 45 (November 16, 2018): 1276–77, https://doi.org/10.15585/mmwr.mm6745a5.

2. Brian A. King et al., "Electronic Cigarette Sales in the United States, 2013–2017," *JAMA* 320, no. 13 (October 2, 2018): 1379–80, https:// doi.org/10.1001/jama.2018.10488.

3. R. A. Miech et al., *Monitoring the Future National Survey Results on Drug Use, 1975–2018*, vol. 1, *Secondary School Students* (Ann Arbor: Institute for Social Research, University of Michigan, 2019), available at http:// monitoringthefuture.org/pubs.html#monographs.

4. Bonnie Herzog, Wells Fargo Securities, LLC, "Wall Street Tobacco Industry Update," February 11, 2019, http://www.natocentral.org/uploads/ Wall_Street_Update_Slide_Deck_February_2019.pdf.

5. Tobacco Products Scientific Advisory Committee, "Menthol Cigarettes and Public Health: Review of the Scientific Evidence and Recommendations" (Silver Spring, MD: US Food and Drug Administration, 2011).

6. Tobacco Control Legal Consortium, "Chicago's Regulation of Menthol Flavored Tobacco Products: A Case Study," 2016, https://www .publichealthlawcenter.org/sites/default/files/resources/tclc-fs-Chicago -Regulation-of-Menthol-Case-Study-Update-2016.pdf.

7. M. Wakefield and G. Giovino, "Teen Penalties for Tobacco Possession, Use, and Purchase: Evidence and Issues," *Tobacco Control* 12, suppl. I (2003): i6–i13, https://tobaccocontrol.bmj.com/content/tobaccocontrol/ 12/suppl_1/i6.full.pdf; L. A. Jason et al., "Youth Tobacco Sales-to-Minors and Possession-Use-Purchase Laws: A Public Health Controversy," *Journal of Drug Education* 35, no. 4 (2005): 275–90.

8. Mary Hrywna et al., "Content Analysis and Key Informant Interviews to Examine Community Response to the Purchase, Possession, and/or Use of Tobacco by Minors," *Journal of Community Health* 29, no. 3 (June 2004):

209–16, https://doi.org/10.1023/B:JOHE.0000022027.03119.38; Wakefield and Giovino, "Teen Penalties"; Alexandra Loukas, Carol Spaulding, and Nell H. Gottlieb, "Examining the Perspectives of Texas Minors Cited for Possession of Tobacco," *Health Promotion Practice* 7, no. 2 (April 1, 2006): 197–205, https://doi.org/10.1177%2F1524839905278852.

9. Tobacco Control Legal Consortium, "Chicago's Regulation," 5.

10. Michael Chaiton et al., "Association of Ontario's Ban on Menthol Cigarettes with Smoking Behavior 1 Month After Implementation," *JAMA Internal Medicine* 178, no. 5 (May 1, 2018): 710–11, https://doi.org/10.1001/jamainternmed.2017.8650.

11. Nick Watts et al., "The *Lancet* Countdown on Health and Climate Change: From 25 Years of Inaction to a Global Transformation for Public Health," *Lancet* 391, no. 10120 (February 10, 2018): 581–630, https://doi.org/10.1016/S0140-6736(17)32464-9.

12. US Global Change Research Program, *Fourth National Climate Assessment*, vol. 2, *Impacts, Risks, and Adaptation in the United States*, ed. D. R. Reidmiller et al. (Washington, DC: US Government Publishing Office, 2018), http://dx.doi.org/10.7930/NCA4.2018.

13. Marshall Burke et al., "Higher Temperatures Increase Suicide Rates in the United States and Mexico," *Nature Climate Change* 8, no. 8 (July 23, 2018): 723–29, https://doi.org/10.1038/s41558-018-0222-x.

14. Andy Haines and Kristie Ebi, "The Imperative for Climate Action to Protect Health," *New England Journal of Medicine* 380, no. 3 (January 17, 2019): 263–73, https://doi.org/10.1056/NEJMra1807873.

15. World Health Organization, *COP24 Special Report: Health and Climate Change* (Geneva: WHO, 2018), https://apps.who.int/iris/bitstream/handle/10665/276405/9789241514972-eng.pdf?ua=1.

16. Stephane Hallegatte et al., *Shock Waves: Managing the Impacts of Climate Change on Poverty* (Washington, DC: World Bank, 2016), https://openknowledge.worldbank.org/handle/10986/22787.

17. World Bank Group, *Climate-Smart Healthcare: Low-Carbon and Resilience Strategies for the Health Sector* (Washington, DC: World Bank, January 1, 2017), http://documents.worldbank.org/curated/en/322251495434571418/pdf/113572-WP-PUBLIC-FINAL-WBG-Climate-smart-Healthcare-002.pdf.

Index

ACA. *See* Affordable Care Act
accreditation, 83–84
Active Transportation Alliance, 96
activism, 41, 183
Addams, Jane, 40–41
advertising
 public service, 12–13, 147–56, 183–84
 tobacco, 140–41, 144–47, 168
Affordable Care Act (ACA), 7, 50, 69, 78, 92, 110, 122
African Americans, 148–50, 166
 health disparities and, 54–56, 151
 menthol cigarettes and, 141, 145–47, 165
Alameda County, California, 86
AllianceChicago, 126
American Public Health Association (APHA), 103–4
American Statistical Association, 29
APHA. *See* American Public Health Association
Arizona, 174
astroturfing, 133–34, 135, 139, 166

Barbot, Oxiris, 181
Berwick, Donald, 122
Big Baby campaign, 155
Big Cities Health Coalition, 96
big data, 8–10, 19, 99, 101–3, 107
 money and, 109
 precision and, 108
 See also data
Big Tobacco, 11, 137–39, 140, 158–59, 166–67, 184.
 See also cigarettes; e-cigarettes; tobacco
Blue Cross Blue Shield of Illinois, 94
Bonner, Thomas Neville, 36
Boston, Massachusetts, 22
breast cancer, 55, 62, 66, 95
Breslow, Lester, 7, 86, 104
Brown & Williamson Tobacco Corporation, 143, 144, 145, 146, 147
Bruhn, John G., 85–86

California, 92, 137, 174, 176, 183
capitalism, 22, 38

carbon dioxide, 175
CCDTR. *See* Chicago Center for Diabetes Translation Research
CDC. *See* Centers for Disease Control and Prevention
CeaseFire. *See* Cure Violence
Centers for Disease Control and Prevention (CDC), 54, 82, 92–93, 107, 185
Charleston, North Carolina, 22
Chesbrough, Ellis Sylvester, 33–34
Chicago, Illinois, history of, 31–32, 52–53
 public health and, 6–7, 33–42
Chicago Center for Diabetes Translation Research (CCDTR), 66
Chicago Clean Indoor Air Ordinance, 158
Chicago Department of Health, 37–38
Chicago Department of Transportation, 94
Chicago Health Atlas, 114–15
Chicago Health Information Technology Regional Extension Center, 106
Chicago Park District, 96
Chicago Relief and Aid Society, 36
Chicago River
 pollution of, 32, 33
 reversal of, 38–39
Chicago Sanitary and Ship Canal, 39
Chi Hack Night, 115–16
cholera, 6, 30–31, 32–33
Christoffel, Katherine, 96–97
cigarettes
 menthol, 141–48, 159, 163–66
 taxes on, 11, 169
 youth marketing of, 140–41, 160, 168
 See also Big Tobacco; e-cigarettes; tobacco
climate change, 173–78, 183
 community health and, 12, 171–72
 cost of, 175–76
 debate over, 138
 poverty and, 176–77
climate-resilient development, 176
climate-smart strategies, 178